Robson Roose

Waste and Repair in modern Life

Robson Roose

Waste and Repair in modern Life

ISBN/EAN: 9783743331082

Manufactured in Europe, USA, Canada, Australia, Japa

Cover: Foto ©ninafisch / pixelio.de

Manufactured and distributed by brebook publishing software (www.brebook.com)

Robson Roose

Waste and Repair in modern Life

CONTENTS.

	PAGE
I. Introduction	1
II. The Wear and Tear of London Life	11
III. Rest and Repair in London Life	34
IV. The Art of Prolonging Life	58
V. Clothing as a Protection Against Cold	94
VI. A Contribution to the Alcohol Question	112
VII. Fasting and its Physiology	144
VIII. The Spread of Diphtheria	163
IX. The Propagation and Prevention of Cholera	187
X. Infection and Disinfection	218
XI. The London Water Supply	272
XII. Health-resorts and their Uses	310
Index	351

I.

INTRODUCTION.

THE Essays collected in this volume were written at frequent intervals during the last ten years; they deal with various subjects relating to Sanitary Science and Public Health —topics always interesting, and perhaps never more so than at the present moment. Various additions and alterations, rendered necessary by the rapid growth of knowledge since these Essays were first published, have been made; but in the arrangement of them no special sequence has been attempted, save that in one or two cases those which treat of kindred themes have been brought together.

It is not, of course, claimed that any of the subjects are exhaustively handled, still less that the volume constitutes a complete treatise on Sanitary Science. The author has aimed at presenting the more important details of a few subjects in an intelligible manner, and at pointing out the lessons to be drawn from each statement. He would be glad to feel that he had caused his readers to take some interest in questions which are of vital importance to all educated persons, not only individually, but also as members of the community, and that he had been enabled to arouse in some minds a desire to become acquainted with the important details of sanitary science. There is no lack of works on Personal and Public Health, written by men thoroughly conversant with the theory and practice of Hygiene, and easily intelligible by any one of ordinary education.

The sanitary legislation of England may be said to date from the passing of the Public Health Act of 1848, but it was not until 1875 that a really comprehensive measure was placed on the Statute Book. Before the passing of the first of these Acts, sanitation was, for the most part, left to the voluntary efforts of individuals, many of whom did good work in certain limited spheres. To go back only as far as the beginning of the last century, we find that the utmost carelessness prevailed, and that no effectual steps were taken to prevent the occurrence of pestilences now happily banished from our shores. The Great Plague in 1665 no doubt suggested lessons which for a time bore good fruit, but the fire in the following year led to results infinitely more valuable than any reformers could have achieved. It abolished many of the conditions under which epidemic diseases had previously flourished.

More than a hundred years after the Great Plague, the lessons taught by that visitation had been to a great extent forgotten. It was not until a private individual had visited, at his own expense, most of the jails in England, that the insanitary and inhuman conditions which prevailed in those centres of infection attracted public attention. It is difficult now to realise that in 1774 the atmosphere of the prisons which John Howard entered was distinctively the atmosphere of typhus, that the prisons were the central seminaries and forcing-houses from which the typhus contagion of those days was ever overflowing into fleets, and barracks, and hospitals, and inspiring a constant terror into courts of justice and the population at large. Howard's labours, and the evidence he gave before a Committee of the House of Commons, were speedily fruitful in results. Changes were gradually made in the sanitary conditions of prisons, and improvement followed improvement. At the present day it must be admitted that a state very near perfection has been arrived at, and that the sanitary excellence of prisons far surpasses that which can be secured for many thousands of honest and well-behaved Englishmen.

The good effected by Howard was not interred with his bones. Not only were prisons reformed, but a new school of action was founded, one which taught that continuous investigation and steady perseverance are imperatively requisite in dealing with grave social evils. The fact that prisons could be rendered as wholesome as the best ordinary dwelling-houses must have been a marvellous revelation to those who had long been cognisant of the evil, but had regarded it as practically irremediable.

Howard's experiences of the conditions under which typhus prevailed led him to adopt accurate ideas of its causation. When he visited the prisons on the Continent he found, to his great surprise, that they were free from fever, although they were no less close, crowded, and impure than our own. He brings the result of his observations and inquiries concerning the cause of the jail-fever to this pointed conclusion: "If it were asked," says he, "what is the cause of the jail-fever, it would in general be readily replied, the want of fresh air and cleanliness; but as I have found, in some prisons abroad, cells and dungeons as offensive and dirty as any I have observed in this country, but in which this distemper was unknown, I am obliged to look out for some additional cause for its production"—which additional cause can be no other than the contagious poison emanating from the bodies of those who have the fever. The disease was not generated within the jails, but, once imported there, it was propagated with terrible rapidity.

The next important discovery in Sanitary Science was that of vaccination, which was first practised by Edward Jenner in 1796. It is needless to describe the circumstances which led to the discovery that by inoculating human beings with matter taken from an eruption on cows, the individuals so treated could be rendered proof against the contagion of small-pox; and, further, that the vaccine virus, when transmitted, by engrafting, from one person to another, retained its protective power. The objections made to the practice, and the controversies with regard to its efficacy are matters of common knowledge, but the general result of all scientific inquiries has been to confirm Jenner's views. It must be allowed that he placed too high an estimate on the protective powers of vaccination. Complete protection, though not always attainable, is certainly the general rule, and it is equally certain that small-pox in vaccinated persons is almost always milder in type and shorter in duration than the same disease among the unvaccinated.

Jenner's explanation of the effects of his method was that the vaccine disease is in reality small-pox, rendered mild by passing through the system of the cow; and this view has been remarkably confirmed by the researches and experiments of Pasteur and others during the last quarter of a century. The sphere of protective inoculation has been enormously enlarged, and there is much ground for hope that, by methods analogous to those of vaccination, immunity may be attained against the attacks of many infectious diseases. In the Essay on "Diphtheria" an account is given of the preparation of the *antitoxin*, with regard to which it may at least be affirmed that its value is distinctly greater than that of any other remedy previously used. The extent of its power cannot as yet be positively estimated, but there is every reason to expect that a more extended trial will only confirm present experience. Other *antitoxins* have been prepared for the treatment of tetanus, cholera, and typhoid fever; but the experiments hitherto made are not sufficient to justify any final conclusion.

If we turn to the progress of Sanitary Legislation, we find that since 1875 many Acts have been passed having for their object the improvement of the public health. The Public Health Act itself has been amended again and again, and laws have been enacted for the regulation of canal boats and other movable dwellings, and of offensive trades, for the sanitation of factories and workshops, the notification and prevention of infectious diseases, the prevention of the pollution of rivers, adulteration of articles of food, and other subjects more or less closely connected with hygiene. All these laws are enormously in advance of any legislation hitherto passed for the protection of the public health. It is scarcely an exaggeration to say that if their administration were perfect, there would be no more insanitary dwellings, no polluted water supply, no accumulation of filth, and no preventable spread of infectious disease in any part of the country. It is in the direction of improved administration and the consolidation and simplification of existing statutes, rather than in any further increase in their volume, that reform is now most needed.

A few words must be added on Personal Hygiene. The recognition of the fact that every community has an interest in the health and strength of individual members, and that concerted action is necessary in order to obtain practical results, even on a small scale, does not imply that individuals are relieved from the responsibility of taking care of themselves. The most elaborate code of laws, administered with the greatest care and strictness, cannot prevent persons from committing a great variety of acts inconsistent with the maintenance of health. Rules for personal hygiene had been current long before codes of public sanitary law had taken shape, and are not now to be deemed superfluous because many of the conditions of life are regulated by local authorities. For a perfect system of hygiene, we must train the body, the intellect and the moral faculties in a perfect and well-balanced order. At the present day our knowledge of hygiene is advancing with rapid strides—in many respects it is already sufficient; and there is no lack of competent teachers and of willing listeners. Much, however, remains to be done before the hope of the sanitary reformer can be realised. When we pass through the over-crowded streets of our poorer districts, and notice the squalid aspect of the inhabitants and the evidences of uncleanliness, poverty, and misery, we are tempted to doubt whether any real progress has been made, and we are forced to make many allowances for the moral defects of those whose lives are passed under such conditions. But there are, happily, other numerous classes, very differently situated, whose fate, as regards health, is largely in their own hands, and whose members may hasten the progress of hygiene by attending to their own health, by inspiring others to follow their example, and by aiding municipal and imperial social improvements. That prevention is better than cure is universally admitted; but the former process is too often neglected, while the latter is frequently unattainable.

II.

THE WEAR AND TEAR OF LONDON LIFE.

"'Why, sir, you find no man, at all intellectual, who is willing to leave London. No, sir, when a man is tired of London, he is tired of life; for there is in London all that life can afford.'"—BOSWELL'S *Life of Johnson.*

THIS opinion was delivered after an experience of forty years of London life, and when the speaker was close upon his seventieth year. Johnson's dogmatism on this, as on other subjects, was based upon deep conviction; he repeatedly dilates on the advantages of London, its pre-eminence over every other place for variety of enjoyments, for comfort, and for intellectual advantages of all kinds. He never so much as hints at the existence of any possible drawback. It may be taken for granted that Johnson's opinion as to the advantages of living in London is tacitly adopted by many classes of persons at the present day, and with good reason. To the ordinary Englishman desirous of enjoyment, or intellectual culture, or of professional success, no other place in the civilised world offers equal facilities for compassing the objects of his desire. Even by people who have no particular aims in view, life out of London is not unfrequently regarded as a kind of vegetative existence. A much more important and numerous class, embracing those who are forced by the nature of their avocations to spend nearly all their time in London, are wont to adopt the same opinion, tempered, perhaps, in many cases by an appreciation of the drawbacks attendant upon their mode of life.

Admitting to the full all the advantages, I propose to consider some of those disadvantages connected with London life which are daily becoming more and more prominent. I shall refer more especially, and from a medical point of view, to those evidences of "wear and tear" which are the direct results of over work, excitement, and anxiety, and which are so often witnessed among statesmen, politicians, and professional men of all classes actively engaged in London. What is the price which so many of them pay for their advantages of position and for their reputation? Besides answering this question, I shall endeavour to point out how some at least of the drawbacks might be obviated.

It is not my intention to reopen the controversy which took place some years ago on the subject of over work. It was asked by Mr. Greg and others whether society at large was really suffering from an amount of work, physical and mental, injurious to the individual, and therefore to the human race. To this question very diverse answers were given. Some authorities said bluntly that in their opinion more ailments arise from idleness or from want of occupation than from over work, and that for one instance of mischief arising from the latter cause, half a dozen might be met with belonging to the former category. Others, again,—probably those who had met with more workers than idlers,—expressed a different and a more guarded opinion; at least with reference to the proportionate influence exercised by two such widely different causes. It cannot, I think, be shown that, provided all proper precautions are taken, mental work even of the hardest kind, and pursued for an almost indefinite period, really injures the nervous system of the individual thus occupied. Indeed, as a matter of fact, it is almost invariably followed by an entirely opposite result. The human body is a machine so constructed that work is a necessity for its continued existence and well-being; the amount of work it is capable of doing is in strict proportion to the power of the mechanism, and while other machines having no power of repair tend to become weaker and worn out by use, the strength and capacity of the nervous and muscular systems of the human body are increased by exercise, provided that the latter is regulated by certain well-known laws. Injurious effects resulting from hard work are almost always traceable to neglect of obvious precautions.

There are of course immense differences among men as regards capacity for performing mental work of any kind. Previous training, constitution, and temperament are potent factors in determining the amount which each is capable of doing. Some men can stand an enormous amount of mental strain without any apparent injury; others, from what may be called, for want of a better term, "weakness of brain," are incapable of anything requiring mental tension. The worst consequences are noticed in people of moderate brain power, who, in the absence of proper training, attempt the performance of severe mental labour. Their case is similar to that of those who suddenly engage in trials of strength and endurance after an insufficient amount of training, and who either exhaust themselves by overtaxing their nervous energies, or induce disorders of the heart or lungs, or strain of some portion of the muscular system, by the violence of their efforts. When a man is being prepared for great muscular exertion, he undergoes a course of training in which the severity of the work assigned to him is gradually and cautiously increased, and the same rule should be adopted for those whose mental powers are about to be severely taxed. If this condition be fulfilled, if a proper amount of sleep can be obtained, and if the appetite remains at its normal level, the brain will bear almost any amount of *steady strain* in the form of severe mental labour.

With regard to health, it is needless to dilate upon the advantages of the combination of health of body with that of mind. Such a combination when it exists cannot be sufficiently prized. The fact, however, remains that not a little of the brain-work of the world is done by men whose standard of health is extremely low; and a weak and ailing condition of body has been proved to be quite compatible with great ability for severe mental exertion. Such cases are, however, the exception; their existence serves to demonstrate the compensatory power existent in the human frame.

Ordinary experience teaches us that monotonous mental toil is far more trying than even a greater amount of work of a diversified character. The same law holds good in respect of bodily labour. When all the muscles are exercised, none are specially fatigued, unless the exercise be immoderate in character. But when only one set of muscles is called into play for lengthened periods, weakness or even partial paralysis is a not unfrequent result. The last point, referring to the effect of anxiety and worry, will be more appropriately considered after I have endeavoured to sketch those features of London life which may be said to necessitate an undue amount of wear and tear. There is little doubt that in many cases it is not the amount of work that is mischievous, but the absence of proper regulations, the attempt to carry on simultaneously several different occupations, and the worry and anxiety which such attempts cannot fail to cause. As evidence of the fact that many men at the present day attempt to live three or four lives at once, I will give a few examples out of many that have come under my notice, taking them from among politicians and the professional classes of the metropolis. There is perhaps little or nothing that is novel in the details I am about to give, but I feel assured that the lessons which may and should be drawn from them are far too much neglected.

I will take for my first sketch the experience of a barrister in good practice. As a general rule, a barrister begins his daily work at his chambers about half-past nine. After a short stay there he passes the next five or six hours in court, either engaged in a case or cases, or waiting for them to come on. While thus waiting he occupies himself with other work— *e.g.*, reading briefs, drawing pleadings, etc. If his attendance be not required in court, he would be working in his chambers, writing opinions, consulting reports and standard authorities in support of such opinions and contentions. Whatever his occupations, he spends but a few minutes over lunch; whether heavy or light it is despatched in the least possible time. His ordinary work detains him at his chambers till seven o'clock, when he goes home to dinner, generally taking with him documents and books to be studied at night. If this were a complete sketch of a barrister's work, it would be absurd to say that any undue amount of wear and tear was necessarily associated therewith. But his legal duties are perhaps the least arduous of those that fall to his lot. As a general rule a barrister, ambitious of rising in his profession, must seek other spheres of activity besides the law-courts. It is almost an absolute necessity that he should enter the House of Commons, and to get there he must expend not a little time and trouble, and make, perhaps, several unsuccessful attempts. As a member he must be in his place at four, or as soon afterwards as he can leave the law-courts. The sittings, of course, vary much in length; even at the present day, important divisions may require the attendance of members till long after midnight. When Parliament rises for the vacation the work of the circuit begins, to be varied in some cases by frequent journeys to London for professional purposes. The work of the Attorney- or Solicitor-General, or of a leading Queen's Counsel, though in some particulars different from that of the ordinary barrister, is quite as continuous. The law officers of the Crown have, of course, much private legal business to transact in addition to the duties, professional and Parliamentary, connected with their offices. Society, moreover, claims a share of the successful barrister's time. Other conditions being favourable, to be seen by the public greatly assists the aspirant to success; and when a good position has been attained, the homage which society demands often involves additional and heavier sacrifices. If to these details of a barrister's work be added his correspondence, private and professional, and the duties connected with his home, family, and friends, it is obvious that his brain and nervous system must be exposed to a strain which, unless due care be taken, and the individual be possessed of an unusual share of mental and bodily vigour, is only too likely to induce serious disorder. As in other cases, the fittest survive, but many drop out of the race. To not a few barristers a robust constitution and a powerful *physique* are of more value than any other qualification.

The duties of a judge, though sufficiently engrossing, are of a less arduous character than those just detailed. A judge's work, heavy as it often is at the present day, is carried on with evenness and regularity, and with little or no excitement. It has, moreover, been preceded by a long course of training; but it can be easily shown that a judge's position is no longer one of dignified ease. In London his duties in court occupy him for five or six hours daily, during which time he must give the closest attention to the evidence and to the arguments of the opposing counsel. He must take notes as a case progresses, and carefully prepare the summing-up for the guidance of the jury. Such a *résumé* is often a perfect model of lucidity and reasoning, and demands the exercise of mental powers of the highest order. Attendance at assizes, the hearing of election petitions, the consideration of appeals and of Crown cases reserved, are the remaining duties which a judge discharges before the public; and if to these be added many social duties which necessarily fall to his share, it must be admitted that the total is sufficient to test to the utmost the fullest vigour both of mind and body.

The daily work of consulting physicians and surgeons in London is scarcely less arduous than that of a barrister, but it is of a more agreeable and far less exciting character. Medical men, too, spend a large portion of their time in their own houses, and the contrast between a physician's study or consulting-room and a barrister's chambers must often attract notice. No one has as yet explained the preference manifested by lawyers (as shown by the state of their chambers) for dust, darkness, and discomforts in general. Such a state of things would not be allowed to exist in an ordinary dwelling-house inhabited by persons claiming to belong to the civilised classes. A consulting physician in London begins his work soon after eight A.M. He probably has a patient or two to visit at that early hour, and on his return will find others waiting who have been allowed to come before the regular consultation hour. Patients continue to arrive, and are seen in turn until the list is exhausted—a process which is sometimes not completed till one or even two o'clock. Then luncheon must be rapidly despatched, and if the physician or surgeon be connected with the large London hospitals, he must, twice a week at least, visit the patients under his care. These visits are always made early in the afternoon, and after this duty is discharged there are private patients to be seen at their own houses, consultations to be held, and, in the case of members of a hospital staff, lectures to be delivered perhaps three or four times a week. Consultations in the country take up more or less of a physician's time; these are usually held in the afternoon. By seven or eight o'clock the work is generally over, so far as attendance on patients is concerned; and after dinner the physician's time is, if he so chooses, at his own disposal. He must, however, keep himself well acquainted with whatever is going on in the medical and scientific world generally. He must therefore devote some time to the medical journals and reviews, and to a perusal of any specially important new book. It generally happens that the evening is the only portion of the day that he can spare for these subjects. Then there are the various medical societies, such as the Medico-Chirurgical, the Medical, the Clinical, etc., meetings of which are held weekly or fortnightly during eight months of the year. Literary labour often makes further demands upon the physician's time; and if he wishes to become popular, he must, like the barrister, pay some attention to the claims of society, and not fail to appear as often as possible at receptions, conversaziones, dinner-parties, etc. A life spent in the manner thus imperfectly sketched has a large share of enjoyment of the best kind: mind and body are kept fully employed, and under favourable conditions at least a fair measure of success is generally attainable. Of course there are drawbacks; at the beginning, and for some years afterwards, the *res angusta domi*, the scarcity of patients, and the necessity for keeping up what are called "appearances," often give rise to very serious forebodings, and middle life is not unfrequently reached before the income is found to balance the expenditure.

A glance at the work imposed upon members of Parliament will suffice to show that it involves no ordinary amount of wear and tear. Work begins in the Committee-rooms at noon; the House assembles at four, and the sittings are often prolonged till midnight. Before the adoption of the twelve o'clock rule, readers of the debates had become quite familiar with the announcement, "The House was still sitting when we went to press"! A newly elected member of Parliament has a great deal to learn before he becomes conversant with his duties, and he is fortunate if he finds time to make himself even moderately well acquainted with the Blue Books, papers, etc., which are annually published. Besides his duties at Westminster, he must attend to his constituents, must show himself among them from time to time, and must be ever ready to listen to complaints, suggestions, or even dictates. The work of a Cabinet Minister varies with the office he fills, the state of public business, and accidental circumstances. He begins the day by making himself acquainted with the contents of the daily papers, and perhaps by giving a few minutes to his private correspondence. The study of official papers, Blue Books, etc., will occupy him till eleven o'clock, the ordinary time of attendance at his office, where he remains until the meeting of the House to which he belongs. The sittings in the House of Lords are generally very short; they rarely last more than an hour or two. In the House of Commons they are only too apt to run to the opposite extreme. In addition to official work, not a few hours are required for preparing Parliamentary speeches and extra-Parliamentary discussions of various kinds. Besides being in constant communication with his secretaries, a Cabinet Minister has frequently to consult various officials, and to grant interviews to those who can show any cause for requesting them. If in charge of any important measure in Parliament, he must be present during every debate upon it, and often make speeches in its support. Replies to questions have to be carefully prepared, assistance being, of course, given by the permanent officials of the department. Attendances at Cabinet Councils and meetings of the Privy Council, at State balls and concerts, at dinners and meetings of every conceivable kind, absorb a large portion of the time unoccupied in Parliamentary work; and if to these items be added the multifarious duties of a private character which almost necessarily devolve upon him, it will be readily admitted that the work of a Cabinet Minister at the present day is such as to tax to the utmost even the highest degrees of mental and physical vigour. The diversified character of his work would appear to be its redeeming feature.

To the ordinary member of the House of Commons, and especially to one who is not as yet hardened by experience, disappointment and a sense of weariness must often make themselves keenly felt. Many a man enters upon Parliamentary life under the idea that he has an important mission to fulfil, but session after session passes and he finds himself no nearer to the goal. Meanwhile he has had to listen night after night to an incessant flow of talk, the larger portion of which is unattended by any practical result. Time and energy are alike misapplied and wasted, and though a powerful and huge machine is at work, the results too often appear practically *nil.* There are at times other reasons for disappointment and disgust. Speeches made and votes given for party purposes in support of measures believed to be mischievous must, in some cases at least, be productive of no ordinary amount of self-contempt.

It may be objected that the instances to which I have referred are of a numerically exceptional character, that these professional classes constitute a small minority of the population, and that the toil in which they are engaged is very different from that which occupies the remainder of the community. It would not be difficult to show that the differences are those of kind rather than of degree. Evidences of work being carried on at high pressure meet us at every turn. I need only refer to the over work in elementary schools, to the "cramming" for competitive examinations, and to the constantly increasing difficulty of the questions as shown by the large number of candidates rejected at public examinations of all kinds. Even in our recreations there are evidences of a similar spirit. In fact, we take pains to turn play itself into work. The best and most popular of our national games, as played during the last few seasons, must often have been anything but a recreation (in the true sense of the word) to those engaged in it. If we turn to commercial life, the same features confront us. What is trade at the present day but competition in its severest forms? Incessant struggles to get on, trampling, crushing, elbowing, and treading on each other's heels, are manifest symptoms of the present phase of industrial progress. He who does not move with the crowd is thrust back by the violence of others who put themselves forward.

To the question whether any penalties are attached to this manner of living only one answer can be given. Every age is characterised by the presence or prevalence of special disorders of health which have a more or less obvious causation. At the present day "want of tone" is the characteristic feature of disorders in general, and in none is it more obvious than in those which peculiarly affect official and professional men working at high pressure. As might be expected, the signs of this "want of tone," or weakening of the nervous system, vary in different persons; but the presence of certain symptoms may be regarded as a test of the actual condition. Of these, sleeplessness is the most important; if allowed to continue, while the individual endeavours to perform his usual tasks, grave disorder of the nervous machinery must soon set in. The restoration of energy, which sleep alone can afford, is necessary for the maintenance of nervous vigour; and whereas the muscular system, if over-taxed, at last refuses to work, the brain under similar circumstances too frequently refuses to rest. The sufferer, instead of trying to remove or lessen the cause of his sleeplessness, comforts himself with the hope that it will soon disappear, or else has recourse to alcohol, morphia, the bromides, chloral, etc. Valuable and necessary as these remedies often are (I refer especially to the drugs), there can be no question as to the mischief which attends their frequent use ; and there is much reason to fear that their employment in the absence of any medical authority is largely on the increase. Many of the "proprietary articles" sold by druggists, and in great demand at the present day, owe their efficacy to one or more of these powerful drugs. Not a few deaths have been caused by their use, and in a still larger number of cases they have helped to produce the fatal result. Sleeplessness is almost always accompanied by indigestion in some one or other of its Protean forms, and the two conditions react upon and aggravate each other. If rest cannot be obtained, and if the vital machine cannot be supplied with a due amount of fuel, and, moreover, fails to utilise that which is supplied, mental and bodily collapse cannot be far distant. The details of the downward process vary, but the result is much the same in all cases. Sleeplessness and loss of appetite are followed by loss of flesh and strength, nervous irritability alternating with depression, palpitation, and other derangements of the heart, especially at night, and many of those symptoms grouped together under the old term, "hypochondriasis." When this stage has been reached, "the borderlands of insanity" are within measurable distance, even if they have not already been reached.

The advocates of what is popularly known as "progress" at the present day will doubtless be surprised at learning (from a distinguished American physician) that the number of the insane is greater in a community in proportion to the political and religious freedom of the population; that is, to the opportunity they enjoy of working out their own purposes, whether in relation to this world or the next, in the manner most agreeable to themselves. The explanation, of course, is that in such communities the causes of insanity are always numerous and widespread. If Dr. Wood's opinion be well founded, the prospect, so far as this country is concerned, must appal those who are already aware of the marked increase of mental disorder. The fact may, perhaps, constitute a weighty argument in favour of more frequent periods of rest, if not of thankfulness. We live in an age when preventive medicine has achieved its greatest triumphs, but the prevention of undue mental strain, of anxiety, excitement, and disappointment consequent upon struggles for power, influence, or wealth cannot be reduced to a system or effected by public authority. Individuals, however, might do something to lessen the wear and tear of modern life. A certain amount of anxiety—the sensation which Dr. Hughlings Jackson has happily described as "fright spread out thin"—is, of course, unavoidable; but a much larger proportion results from circumstances for the most part really under our own control, but which we strive to exaggerate and multiply. Many a man might ask himself whether the game he is playing is really worth the candle, and whether less bustle and hurry, or even one of the quieter walks of life, would not, after all, be much more conducive to happiness than a constant whirl of excitement and anxiety. There is no exaggeration in Mr. Greg's remark that "a life without leisure and without pause—a life of haste and excitement—a life so full that we have no time to reflect where we have been and where we intend to go, what we have done and what we plan to do, can scarcely be deemed an adequate or worthy life."

Such is the life led by far too many at the present day, and its effects are only too manifest. One effect of this high-pressure existence is that it leaves even the successful man who has gained much to retire *upon*, nothing to retire *to*; for literature, science, domestic ties, philanthropic interests, nature itself, have all been neglected and lost sight of during the mad rush and struggle of the last thirty years, and these are treasures the key to which soon grows rusty, and friends once slighted cannot be called back at will. It is, after all, nothing to the purpose to say that more mischief is caused by idleness than by excessive work. Idleness is an evil, and deserves to be punished; work is, or ought to be, a blessing. But is there no middle course between dull stagnation and those results of excessive pressure which Mr. Gladstone has termed " moral dissipation?" Perhaps one of the worst features of the present day is the contempt for that *aurea mediocritas* which, always praised but rarely pursued, is yet assuredly not beyond the reach of those who make it their ideal.

III.

REST AND REPAIR IN LONDON LIFE.

BY way of supplementing my remarks on the wear and tear of London life, I propose to offer a few suggestions as to the means whereby these evils might be moderated or lessened. I do not pretend to say that I know of any agent capable of arresting that constant expenditure of energy which results from the proper employment of our faculties. Life involves incessant change, and even decay itself is a manifestation of energy of a certain kind. Waste is harmful only when it is excessive and not speedily followed by processes of repair, and to arrest normal change would be to check the expression of life, or even to cause death. What I do maintain is, that while health is incomparably the greatest blessing vouchsafed to man, here, in London, many of the conditions under which a constantly increasing number live, militate against its attainment, and by so doing diminish the happiness and add to the sorrows of those who ought to be able to choose between good and evil. I alluded to "want of tone" as a striking peculiarity of many of our common ailments, and by means of a few illustrations I sought to demonstrate some of the causes which tended to produce this condition. The more important of these may be thus briefly summarised: excessive and persistent brain-work without sufficient rest; brain-work in persons incapable by nature, or by reason of imperfect training; the endeavour to carry on simultaneously several occupations; and lastly, over-anxiety and worry connected with daily life, striving after success, disappointed hopes, etc.

The discovery of the cause or causes is a necessary preliminary to the prevention of a given evil. If, on being discovered, such causes are removed, their effects will cease to be displayed. How, it may well be asked, are such causes as those I have just mentioned to be got rid of? Their existence is but too manifest; is their removal possible? I believe that with regard to some of them the question might be answered in the affirmative, and that in the case of others their effects might be considerably lessened by the adoption of a few precautionary measures. It appears to me that the responsibility for their widespread existence must be shared by the State, by society in general, and by those individuals who are the principal sufferers. If this statement be correct, it is surely worth while to inquire what amount of amelioration each of the parties concerned may be asked to contribute. I shall be very brief in my remarks as to the State and society in general, inasmuch as little or nothing in the way of reform can be expected from either of these; the important points for consideration are the measures which individuals might adopt so as to prevent or mitigate "wear and tear," and to combat their untoward results when once developed.

That the State is responsible for a large amount of unnecessary wear and tear cannot, I think, be denied; I will refer to only one of the conditions of modern political life—viz., the management of business in the House of

Commons. This, at the present day, is such, that diligent attendance during a single Session is sufficient to wear out the physical and mental powers of the strongest man. The late hours, the long sittings, the frivolous questionings, the weariness and emptiness of many of the debates, furnish an ample explanation of the want of tone and ill-health of many of those who endeavour to do their duty. It cannot be said that these evils are necessary. With regard to the expenditure of time, is it not possible to devise some means whereby the daily work could be got through, say in six hours at the outside? Would less real work be done if the House of Commons were to meet at half-past four and never sit later than twelve, and if the business were adapted to the time, and not the time to the business? The practicability of this alteration has been proved by its adoption as a general rule.

In regard to the responsibility of society for much of the wear and tear of the present day, and to any improvement which can be obtained at the hands of that all-powerful body, it will be difficult to offer any practical suggestions. In a criticism on my previous paper, the *Spectator* asserts that the endurance of the racket of society is altogether voluntary, and infers therefore that it could be dispensed with. No doubt it is voluntary in the simple meaning of the term; but the obligation to pay court to society is one which cannot be evaded with impunity by those who wish to rise. Disagreeable as the notion may be, it is nevertheless true that being seen in society is often as useful to the professional man as advertising is to the tradesman. "Out of sight, out of mind," holds good in both cases, and in that of the former an increased measure of success is followed by more imperious demands on the part of society. If advantages are to be retained, their possessor must show that he is able to bear the popular gaze, and the exhibition flatters those whose support will tend to bring further successes within reach. If society-haunting afforded the necessary relaxation to the over-worked brain, it might be excused on that ground; but unfortunately a heavy price is often paid by men who give to society the time which ought to be devoted to rest or relaxation. It is curious that on the other side of the

Atlantic the claims of society are found to exercise an injurious influence on a very different class. We have lately been told that ill-health from over work among American children is attributable not to school-pressure, but to parental ambition and to the " society engagements " of the pupils.

In a primitive state of society the more important of the laws of health are unconsciously obeyed; but this passive condition of obedience is not possible for the active workers in large cities. They are surrounded by unfavourable circumstances, so common as to be little noticed, and often considered as practically unavoidable even by those who regard them as evils. In the case of individuals the problem which offers itself for solution is twofold—viz., how to lessen the causes which induce excessive wear and tear; and having done all that seems possible in this respect, how to preserve health under those unfavourable conditions which are, or appear to be, irremovable.

In estimating the amount and character of brain-work which can be performed without causing undue wear and tear, it is obvious that no rules of universal applicability can be laid down. Men's capacities for work differ as much as their features, and very much depends upon previous training; but a few practical suggestions may not be without value. In my former paper I mentioned two important tests, by the aid of which it could be determined in any given case whether hard mental toil was producing mischief or not: one of these is capacity for sleep, and the second, of subordinate though nearly equal value, the state of the appetite and digestion. If the sleep be normal in amount and refreshing in character, and if the appetite and digestion remain good, it is certain that no harm is being done. With regard to the quantity of sleep, it is impossible to lay down any hard and fast rule, but six or seven hours are generally sufficient. There is probably some truth in the old maxim that an hour's sleep before midnight is equal in value to two hours afterwards, if only because its adoption encourages early hours. The great value of rest as a restorative agent is clearly shown by the fact that a capacity for long, refreshing sleep is regarded by surgeons as considerably lessening the risks of an operation, especially one entailing much shock or prolonged repair. It is also a matter of common experience that persons who sleep soundly and drop off to sleep easily are capable of sustaining a larger amount of mental and corporeal exertion than those who find it difficult to get to sleep, and who wake up several times during the night. Shakespeare recommends as safe counsellors men "such as sleep o' nights."

There is much difference of opinion concerning the desirability of an after-dinner nap. Those who advocate it cite the example of animals; but these gorge themselves with food whenever opportunity offers, and are heavy and drowsy in consequence. A short rest is, however, different from lethargic sleep, and often appears to do good. Brain-work should certainly be forbidden after dinner; the interval between it and bed-time should be devoted to recreation and amusement. In the case of elderly people a short nap after a late dinner often aids digestion; but as a general rule it is better for such persons to make their principal meal at 2 P.M. The digestive powers of most elderly people are at a low ebb in the evening. When sleeplessness is troublesome, relief should be sought for in the discovery and removal of the cause, whenever possible. The condition is often due to indigestion, and when this is the case, the ordinary remedies for inducing sleep are worse than useless. The nervous relations between the brain and the stomach are so intimate, that disorder of the one organ is almost certain to affect the other. Excitement, worry, and anxiety, which have their seat in the brain, interfere with the functions of the stomach, and in like manner anything that unduly taxes the power of, or irritates the stomach, disorders the circulation and nutrition of the brain. The sleeplessness often complained of by gouty persons is due to the poisonous effect of the morbid material upon the nervous system. Excessive smoking, too much alcohol, tea, and coffee, often resorted to by over-worked persons, are frequent causes of sleeplessness. In all these cases the cause is removable, while the effect may be counteracted by appropriate treatment. Nothing is more mischievous, however, than to continue the habits, and to have recourse to drugs to combat the effects. A due amount of exercise tends to induce normal sleep, and such exercise need not be of a violent character. A walk of two or three miles daily is sufficient, and is perhaps as much as a busy man can find time for. A ride on horseback—the Palmerstonian cure for gout—is probably the best form of exercise for those whose minds are constantly at work. It has been well said that a man must come out of himself when in the saddle; he is forced to attend to his horse and to notice the objects he meets. Walking may be a merely automatic process, and afford little, if any, relief to the mind; and carriage exercise may be practically valueless, if the mind is not diverted from what had previously occupied it.

Most people allow that early rising is advantageous, but there are, it is to be feared, comparatively few brain-workers who adopt the habit. They allege, and with some reason, that they can work best at night, because the surroundings are quiet and there is freedom from disturbance. When they state, however, that they themselves feel better fitted for work, they are, as a general rule, misinterpreting their own sensations. They feel quiet because they are tired; one part seems fit for work because the other is too weary to protest. A recourse to tea, coffee, or alcohol helps the mind for a time, but the effect of these *stimuli* upon the wearied organism is only to increase the penalty that must sooner or later be paid, in the form of sleeplessness and other evidences of nervous disturbance. Morning is the time for work; after a due amount of sleep the mind is more fitted to grapple with difficulties than after a long and fatiguing day. To those unaccustomed to the habit, a strong effort is necessary in order to begin the practice of early rising, and in winter the difficulties would doubtless seem great. Thanks, however, to modern contrivances, a small room can soon be made comfortably warm, and a cup of coffee can be prepared with a minimum of trouble. A man who has done two hours' good work before breakfast feels that he is, to that extent at least, in advance of the majority of his fellow-workers. Dean Hook, we are told by his biographer, considered his morning very short if he did not get to work before half-past five o'clock.

The state of the digestion has been alluded to as a test of the effect which severe mental work is producing on the system. A man who works hard with his brain must eat a sufficient quantity of food to supply the waste of the nervous tissues. Indigestion with its host of troubles is to be kept at bay, and it is often difficult to accomplish this object. Given, however, a fair constitution, much may be done by ordinary care and forethought. A good appetite for breakfast is an excellent test of the state of the digestion and of the good effects of the night's rest. Captain Dalgetty's plan of securing, on all occasions which offer, "as much vivers as the magazine can possibly hold," is not one to be recommended for ordinary persons engaged in peaceable occupations, but there can be no doubt as to the advantage of taking in a reasonable supply before beginning the more arduous labours of the day. The lateness of the dinner hour at the present day necessitates, for most people, a tolerably substantial meal between one and two o'clock; and if a man is kept hard at work during the afternoon, it is highly desirable that he should take at least half an hour's rest before dinner. Nothing is more likely to produce indigestion than to eat even moderately when mind and body are thoroughly wearied with the day's toil.

Judging from the enormous number of remedies for indigestion which are being offered to the public, and from the lavish manner in which they are advertised, it would appear that the disorder must be a very common one, and that the remedies supply a want which is urgently felt. In no other country in Europe is there the same profusion of nostrums, and the reason for this difference is perhaps not far to seek. In former days men's stomachs were often overtaxed by too much food; at present excessive eating is out of fashion, but the digestive organs of many persons are unequal to the task which they are called upon to fulfil. Brain-workers are notoriously prone to suffer from indigestion, some of the causes of which have been already indicated. The fact is that the process of digestion, even of suitable food, makes a considerable, though unfelt, demand upon the nervous energy of the system. If too much of this energy has been expended in other ways, or is diverted, when most required, into other channels, digestion will be more or less imperfect. Take the case of a man who, after a hard day's work, sits down to dinner at eight or half-past, having taken a hasty and scanty lunch some hours previously. His sensations tell him that he is terribly in want of food, but they do not warn him that he has little or no power of digestion left. He eats freely and rapidly, and one form of discomfort is soon exchanged for another. Digestion goes on very slowly, and the process is far from complete when bedtime comes. The sufferer is weary, but sleep is unrefreshing, and probably broken by dreams or nightmare. He begins the succeeding day weighted with the burdens of its predecessor. Now all these evils—and they are no slight ones to the man obliged to work hard with his brains—might be prevented by a little forethought. The dinner hour at the present day is far too late; it would seem that we dine when we are literally unable to do anything else. Seven o'clock is quite late enough; and if that be the fixed hour, a certain time ought to be set apart for luncheon. Then, again, a man who feels exhausted for want of food should eat sparingly, and above all things slowly. The suggestion I have already made, of half an hour's rest before dinner, would, if adopted, avert many of the troubles which are caused by taking food when the stock of nervous energy necessary for digestion has been well-nigh exhausted.

With regard to the quality and kind of food best suited to men who are working hard with their brains, space will not allow me to offer more than a few suggestions. A man must be very unobservant or very foolish if he does not find out for himself what suits him and what does not; but few men realise the extent to which our sensations are influenced by the condition of our digestive organs, and what an effect indigestion often produces upon our views of things in general, and our own prospects in particular. Under any circumstances, if indigestion is to be avoided, a positive sense of satiety should never be experienced after any meal, for this is beyond the point of healthful indulgence, and really signifies that too much has been taken. That which ought to be attained occurs immediately previous to this, and is characterised by ease and quiescence. Much improvement has been effected of late in our methods of preparing food, but a great deal remains to be done in this direction. The increased use of vegetables and of fish as an article of diet is a salutary change, combined as it often is with a diminished consumption of meat. The movement in favour of great moderation in the use of wine and other alcoholic liquors is also bearing good fruit, though no objection can be raised against the lighter wines, especially if diluted with hot water or some one or other of the aerated waters. The taking of a large amount of fluid with meals, however, should be avoided; it is apt to become a habit, and is liable to cause and aggravate indigestion. Iced water is not suitable as a drink at mealtimes. Its habitual use is one of the causes of indigestion, which appears to be endemic in all American cities. With many brainworkers a little alcohol taken with food decidedly aids digestion, but its use must always be followed by rest and not by renewed efforts. The brain is still weary, but the alcohol prevents the weariness from being felt. It is always mischievous to take alcohol between meals in order to stimulate the flagging powers.

Fresh air, recreation of all kinds, and change of scene are the next most important agents for preventing wear and tear and for removing their effects. I shall only add a few words on these subjects. Under the first I would include ventilation; for though most of us appreciate fresh air out of doors, there is far too little attention paid to the renewal of the air in our dwelling-houses, and not a little discomfort results from this neglect. Windows cannot be always kept open, and the problem of ventilation without draught is no doubt difficult of solution. Tobin's contrivances for the admission of fresh air are about the best that have been devised; and the simpler form, that of openings in the window sashes, through which the air is projected upwards and then descends, can be adopted in any room. There should of course be outlets for foul air, and the products of combustion, wherever gas is used. A great reformation is needed in this respect ; in crowded rooms the evil is often very perceptible.

I can only just glance at the subject of recreation, though it is a very important means of repair. The term includes a great variety of measures, and even of employments. Change of work is one form of recreation, because, it may be presumed, the new employment occupies a different portion of the brain, and the one that has worked obtains rest. Monotony of occupation is always irksome, no doubt because certain portions of the brain are exclusively occupied. A hard-worked man should think no form of recreation beneath his notice ; he is fortunate if he has a really satisfactory hobby or two. Talleyrand's prognostication of the kind of old age that awaited the man who did not know whist is full of truth, if it be applied to amusements and hobbies in general. Perhaps its author would scarcely have recommended whist for an old man had he been able to foresee the bewildering modifications which have been made in the way of playing the game. In this, as in other things, the tendency is to turn play into work. Let us hope, however, that some of our simpler forms of recreation may be permitted to survive at least for our time. Books remain, and we may be thankful for the stock we already possess. Reading offers the most available means of recreation. Dean Hook's practice in this respect also is worthy of adoption. He tells us himself that he always had a novel in hand. It lasted him a long time, "but when a man has much to do, a little time thus spent does the mind good." Books, however, should be suited to the occasion. As Bulwer tells us, "when taken indiscriminately, they are no cure for the diseases and afflictions of the mind. There is a world of science necessary in the taking them. I have known some people in great sorrow fly to a novel or the last light book in fashion. One might as well take a rose-draught for the plague. Light reading does not do when the heart is really heavy." By all means let the recreation be conformable to the tastes of the individual, and adapted to his condition. When a man over sixty, who has led a sedentary life, suddenly and vehemently takes to tricycling, he may feel pretty sure that he has failed to catch the meaning of the term "recreation," and that a very different process will certainly develop itself.

The last point for consideration is that which refers to change of scene and holidays. No doubt much of the value of health-resorts is due to the change of scene which is connected with them, though other factors cooperate in the production of the good effects. A hard-worked man, compelled to live in London for many months in the year, confidently expects to receive the greatest benefit from a sojourn at the seaside, or among woods and green fields; and some men while working in London have endeavoured to get as much fresh air as possible by spending their nights at least in the country. Such a plan, unfortunately, seldom, if ever, succeeds; most men who try it soon become aware of its drawbacks. To get really fresh country air, uncontaminated by the smoke of London, one must go at least a dozen miles from the metropolis, and to do this daily, necessitates a double railway journey, besides the drives to and from the stations. The man whose business in London begins at ten, and is over by four or five o'clock, may live twenty miles from his office, but the professional man, with longer and less definite hours of work, does better by keeping close to his post. He ought, however, to avail himself of every opportunity of getting a short change in the country, or at the seaside, at some one or other of the many suitable places within easy reach, such as Brighton, Margate, Seaford, Eastbourne, and the rest. It must be admitted that there is some difficulty in finding comfortable quarters for such short holidays as from Saturday to Monday. Lodging-house keepers do not lay themselves out for visitors of this kind, and hotels are for the most part uncomfortable places, especially on the days mentioned. Those who could afford it would do well to rent a small cottage in the country, which would serve as a retreat whenever a holiday could be obtained. In the number of health-resorts within easy reach, the hard-worked Londoner is exceptionally fortunate as compared with the dwellers in most continental capitals. An occasional change and rest, if only for thirty-six hours, in pure air, would help many a man to get through months of hard work with ease and satisfaction. Even from a money point of view, to be always "up to the mark" would to many men be equivalent to a considerable addition to their income.

The subject of an annual holiday is the last to which I shall refer; there can be no doubt as to the advantages of this means of rest and recreation. Where to spend a holiday and how best to enjoy it are topics which should frequently engage the thoughts of a man who is working at high pressure. The idea of a holiday, even if the realisation be somewhat distant, lessens present discomforts, and the carrying out of a well-devised plan enhances the enjoyment when the time arrives. The number of ways in which a holiday may be profitably spent is almost infinite. Yachting, boating, fishing, etc., will suit those who require bodily rest; while walking, riding, and other forms of active exercise will suggest themselves to a different class. A drive through several English counties, with leisurely visits to all places of interest, might serve as a very pleasant occupation for five or six weeks.

Something definite should be aimed at and done during each holiday; an active-minded man must have occupation of some kind even in his hours of recreation. A change of work is indeed a form of rest, and happily there is no lack of subjects for every variety of mind. While enjoying the fresh air of the seaside, the professional man can prosecute some branch of natural science for which he has a liking, or can indulge in a course of his favourite authors; when travelling abroad, the language of the country, its history, and works of art will afford an ample field both for recreation and pleasant employment. By such means as these, mind and body are alike renewed and invigorated.

I have thus described the principal measures which we ought to take if we wish to reduce to a minimum the wear and tear of London life. They may be briefly described as "rest and repair," and their adoption to a greater or less extent is within the power of most men. I am far from advocating any undue anxiety or unnecessary care with regard to health, but seeing as I do many instances of men breaking down under hard work, and in some cases never regaining their previous condition, I have been led to offer these few remarks by way of advice and warning. If over work and worry cannot be lessened, common sense tells us that we should endeavour to mitigate their effects in every possible way, and the best method of compassing this object is to preserve the mind and body in such a condition as will enable them to perform satisfactorily every function which can reasonably be required of them. If this result cannot be attained, the question of reducing the amount of work will demand a prompt solution. The acquirement of fame and fortune is but a sorry exchange for health and vigour. *Non est vivere, sed valere vita.*

IV.

THE ART OF PROLONGING LIFE.

THE doctrine that a short life is a sign of divine favour has never been accepted by the majority of mankind. Philosophers have vied with each other in depicting the evils and miseries incidental to existence, and the truth of their descriptions has often been sorrowfully admitted, but they have failed to dislodge, or even seriously diminish, that desire for long life which has been deeply implanted within the hearts of men. The question whether life be worth living has been decided by a majority far too great to admit of any doubt upon the subject, and the voices of those who would fain reply in the negative are drowned amid the chorus of assent. Longevity, indeed, has come to be regarded as one of the grand prizes of human existence, and reason has again and again suggested the inquiry whether care or skill can increase the chances of acquiring it, and can make old age, when granted, as comfortable and happy as any other stage of our existence.

From very early times the art of prolonging life, and the subject of longevity, have engaged the attention of thinkers and essayists; and some may perhaps contend that these topics, admittedly full of interest, have been thoroughly exhausted. It is true that the art in question has long been recognised and practised, but the science upon which it really depends is of quite modern origin. New facts connected with longevity have, moreover, been collected within the last few years, and some of these I propose to examine, and further to inquire whether they teach us any fresh means whereby life may be maintained and prolonged.

But before entering upon the immediate subject, there are several preliminary questions which demand a brief examination, and the first that suggests itself is, What is the natural duration of human life? This oft-repeated question has received many different answers; and inquiry has been stimulated by scepticism as to their truth. The late Sir George Cornewall Lewis expressed the opinion that one hundred years must be regarded as a limit which very few, if indeed any, human beings succeed in reaching, and he supported this view by several cogent reasons. He pointed out that almost all the alleged instances of abnormal longevity occurred among the humbler classes, and that it was difficult, if not impossible, to obtain any exact information as to the date of birth and to identify the individuals with any written statements that might be forthcoming. He laid particular stress upon the fact that similar instances were altogether absent among the higher classes, with regard to whom trustworthy documentary evidence was almost always obtainable. He thought that the higher the rank the more favourable would the conditions be for the attainment of a long life. In this latter supposition, however, Sir George Lewis was probably mistaken: the comforts and luxuries appertaining to wealth and high social rank are too often counterbalanced by cares and anxieties, and by modes of living inconsistent with the maintenance of health, and therefore with the prolongation of life. In the introduction to his work on "Human Longevity," Easton says, "It is not the rich or great . . . that become old, but such as use much exercise, are exposed to the fresh air, and whose food is plain and moderate—as farmers, gardeners, fishermen, labourers, soldiers, and such men as perhaps never employed their thoughts on the means used to promote longevity."

The French naturalist, Buffon, believed that if accidental causes could be excluded, the normal duration of human life would be between ninety and one hundred years, and he suggested that it might be measured (in animals as well as in man) by the period of growth to which it stood in a certain proportion. He imagined that every animal might live for six or seven times as many years as were requisite for the completion of its growth. But this calculation is not in harmony with facts, so far, at least, as man is concerned. His period of growth cannot be estimated at less than twenty years; and if we take the lower of the two multipliers, we get a number which, in the light of modern evidence, cannot be accepted as attainable. If the period of growth be multiplied by five, the result will in all probability not be far from the truth.

If we seek historical evidence, and from it attempt to discover the extreme limit of human life, we are puzzled at the differences in the ages said to have been attained. The longevity of the antediluvian patriarchs when contrasted with our modern experience seems incredible. When we look at an individual, say 90 years of age, taking even the most favourable specimen, a prolongation of life to ten times that number of years would appear too absurd even to dream about. There is certainly no physiological reason why the ages assigned to the patriarchs should not have been attained, and it is useless to discuss the subject, for we know very little of the conditions under which they lived. It is interesting to notice that after the Flood there was a gradual decrease in the duration of life. Abraham is recorded to have died at 175; Joshua, some five hundred years later, "waxed old and stricken in age" shortly before his death at 110 years; and his predecessor, Moses, to whom 120 years are assigned, is believed to have estimated the life of man at threescore years and ten—a measure nowadays pretty generally accepted.

There is no reason for believing that the extreme limit of human life in the time of the Greeks and Romans differed materially from that which agrees with modern experience. Stories of the attainment of such ages as 120 years and upwards may be placed in the same category as the reputed longevity of Henry Jenkins, Thomas Parr, Lady Desmond, and a host of others. With regard to later times, such as the Middle Ages, there are no precise data upon which any statements can be based, but there is every reason to believe that the *average* duration of life was decidedly less than it is at present. The extreme limit, indeed, three or four centuries ago, would appear to have been much lower than it is in the nineteenth century. At the request of Mr. Thoms, Sir J. Duffus Hardy investigated the subject of the longevity of man in the thirteenth, fourteenth, fifteenth, and sixteenth centuries, and his researches led him to believe that persons seldom reached the age of 80. He never met with a trustworthy record of a person who exceeded that age.

To bring the investigation down to quite recent times, I cannot do better than utilise the researches of the late Sir G. M. Humphry, Professor of Surgery at Cambridge. In 1886 he obtained particulars relating to fifty-two individuals then living and said to be 100 years old and upwards. The oldest among them claimed to be 108, the next 106, while the average amounted to a little more than 102 years. Many interesting facts connected with the habits and mode of life of these individuals were obtained by Dr. Humphry, and will be referred to in subsequent paragraphs.

A short account of the experience of a few life-assurance companies will conclude this part of my subject. Mr. Thoms tells us that down to 1872 the records of the companies showed that one death among the assured had occurred at 103, one in the 100th, and three in the 99th year. The experience of the National Debt Office, according to the same authority, gave two cases in which the evidence could be regarded as perfect; one of these died in the 102nd year, and the other had just completed that number. In the tables published by the Institute of Actuaries, and giving the mortality experience down to 1863 of twenty life assurance companies, the highest age at death is recorded as 99, and I am informed by the manager of the North British Life Office in Edinburgh, that from 1863 onwards that age had not been exceeded in his experience. In the valuation schedules, which show the highest ages of existing lives in various offices, the ages range from 92 to 95. It is true that one office which has a large business among the industrial classes reports lives at 103, and in one instance at 107; but it must be remembered that among those classes the ages are not nearly so well authenticated as among those who assure for substantial sums. There is, moreover, another source of error connected with the valuation schedules. When a given life is not considered to be equal to the average, a certain number of years is added to the age, and the premium is charged at the age which results from this addition. It follows, therefore, that in some cases the ages given in the schedules are greater by some years than they really are.

Taking into consideration the facts thus rapidly passed under review, it must, I think, be admitted that the natural limit of human existence is that assigned to it in the book of Ecclesiasticus, "The number of a man's days at the most are an hundred years" (chap. xviii. 9). In a very small number of cases this limit is exceeded, but only by a very few years. Mr. Thoms' investigations conclusively show that trustworthy evidence of 110 years having been reached is altogether absent. Future generations will be able to verify or reject statements in all alleged cases of longevity. It must be remembered that previous to the year 1836 there was no registration of births, but only of baptisms, and that the registers were kept in the churches, and contained only the names of those therein baptized.

Whatever number of years may be taken as representing the natural term of human life, whether threescore-and-ten or a century be regarded as such, we are confronted by the fact that only one-fourth of our population attains the former age, and that only about fifteen in 100,000 become centenarians. It is beyond the scope of this article to discuss the causes of premature mortality, but the conditions favourable to longevity, and the causes to which length of days has been assigned, are closely connected with its subject.

A capability of attaining old age is very often handed down from one generation to another, and heredity is probably the most powerful factor in connection with longevity. A necessary condition of reaching advanced age is the possession of sound bodily organs, and such an endowment is eminently capable of transmission. Instances of longevity characterising several generations are frequently brought to notice. A recent and most interesting example of transmitted longevity was that of the veteran guardian of the public health, the late Sir Edwin Chadwick, who, when entertained at a public dinner on the occasion of his reaching his 90th year, informed his entertainers that his father died at the age of 84, his grandfather at 95, and that two more remote ancestors were centenarians.

It is difficult to estimate the influence of other contingencies which affect longevity. With regard to sex, Hufeland's opinion was that women were more likely than men to become old, but that instances of extreme longevity were more frequent among men.

This opinion is to some extent borne out by Dr. Humphry's statistics: of his fifty-two centenarians, thirty-six were women. Marriage would appear to be conducive to longevity. A well-known French *savant*, Dr. Bertillon, states that a bachelor of 25 is not a better life than a married man of 45; and he attributes the difference in favour of married people to the fact that they take more care of themselves, and lead more regular lives, than those who have no such tie. It must, however, be remembered that the mere fact of marrying indicates superior vitality and vigour, and the ranks of the unmarried are largely filled by the physically unfit.

In considering occupations as they are likely to affect longevity, those which obviously tend to shorten life need not be considered. With respect to the learned professions, it would appear that among the clergy the average of life is beyond that of any similar class. It is improbable that this average will be maintained for the future: the duties and anxieties imposed upon the clergy of the present generation place them in a very different position from that of their predecessors. Among lawyers, there have been several eminent judges who attained a great age, and the rank and file of the profession are also characterised by a decided tendency to longevity. The medical profession supplies but few instances of extreme old age, and the average duration of life among its members is decidedly low, a fact which can easily be accounted for: broken rest, hard work, anxieties, exposure to weather and to the risks of infection cannot fail to exert an injurious influence upon health. No definite conclusions can be arrived at with regard to the average longevity of literary and scientific men, but it might be supposed that those among them who are not harassed by anxieties and enjoy fair health would probably reach old age. As a general rule, the duration of life is not shortened by literary pursuits. A man may worry himself to death over his books, or, when tired of them, may seek recreation in pursuits destructive to health; but application to literary work tends to produce cheerfulness, and to prolong rather than shorten the life even of an infirm man. In Professor Humphry's "Report on Aged Persons," containing an account of 824 individuals of both sexes, and between the ages of 80 and 100, it is stated that 48 per cent. were poor, 42 per cent. were in comfortable circumstances, and only 10 per cent. were described as being in affluent circumstances. Dr. Humphry points out that these ratios "must not be regarded as representing the relations of poverty and affluence to longevity, because, in the first place, the poor at all ages and in all districts bear a large proportion to the affluent; and, secondly, the returns are largely made from the lower and middle classes, and in many instances from the inmates of union-workhouses, where a good number of aged people are found." It must also be noticed that the "past life-history" of these individuals showed that the greater proportion (55 per cent.) "had lived in comfortable circumstances," and that only 35 per cent. had been poor.

Merely to enumerate the causes to which longevity has been attributed in attempting to account for individual cases would be a task of some magnitude; it will be sufficient to mention a few somewhat probable theories. Moderation in eating and drinking is often declared to be a cause of longevity, and the assertion is fully corroborated by Dr. Humphry's inquiries. Of his fifty-two centenarians, twelve were recorded as total abstainers from alcoholic drinks throughout life, or for long periods; twenty had taken very little alcohol; eight were reported as moderate in their use of it; and only three habitually indulged in it. It is quite true that a few persons who must be classified as drunkards live to be very old; but these are exceptions to the general rule, and such cases appear to be more frequent than they really are, because they are often brought to notice by those who find encouragement from such examples. The habit of temperance in food, good powers of digestion, and soundness of sleep are other main characteristics of most of those who attain advanced years, and may be regarded as causes of longevity. Not a few old persons are found on inquiry to take credit to themselves for their own condition, and to attribute it to some remarkable peculiarity in their habits or mode of life. It is said that Lord Mansfield, who reached the age of 89, was wont to inquire into the habits of life of all aged witnesses who appeared before him, and that only in one habit, namely, that of early rising, was there any general concurrence. Health is doubtless often promoted by early rising, but the habit is not necessarily conducive to longevity. It is, as Sir H. Holland points out, more probable that the vigour of the individuals maintains the habit than that the latter alone maintains the vitality.

If we pass from probable to improbable causes of longevity, we are confronted by many extravagant assumptions. Thus, to take only a few examples, the immoderate use of sugar has been regarded not only as a panacea, but as decidedly conducive to length of days. Dr. Slare, a physician of the last century, has recorded the case of a centenarian who used to mix sugar with all his food, and the doctor himself was so convinced of the "balsamic virtue" of this substance that he adopted the practice, and boasted of his health and strength in his old age. Another member of the same profession used to take daily doses of tannin (the substance employed to harden and preserve leather), under the impression that the tissues of the body would be thereby protected from decay. His life was protracted beyond the ordinary span, but it is questionable whether the tannin acted in the desired direction. Lord Combermere thought that his good health and advanced years were due, in part at least, to the fact that he always wore a tight belt round his waist. His lordship's appetite was doubtless thereby kept within bounds; we are further told that he was very moderate in the use of all fluids as drink. Cleanliness might be supposed to aid in prolonging life; yet a Mrs. Lewson, who died in the early part of this century, aged 106, must have been a singularly dirty person, We are told that instead of washing she smeared her face with lard, and asserted that " people who washed always caught cold." This lady, no doubt, was fully persuaded that she had discovered the universal medicine.

Many of the alchemists attributed the power of prolonging life to certain preparations of gold, probably under the idea that the permanence of the metal might be imparted to the human system. Descartes is said to have favoured such opinions: he told Sir Kenelm Digby that although he would not venture to promise immortality, he was certain that his life might be lengthened to the period of that enjoyed by the patriarchs. His plan, however, seems to have been the very rational and simple one of checking all excesses and enjoining punctual and frugal meals.

Having thus endeavoured to show the extent to which human life may be prolonged, and having examined some of the causes or antecedents of longevity, the last subject for inquiry is the means by which it may be attained. Certain preliminary conditions are obviously requisite; in the first place there must be a sound constitution derived from healthy ancestors, and in the second there must be a freedom from organic disease of important organs. Given an individual who has reached the "grand climacteric," or threescore-and-three, and in whom these two conditions are fulfilled, the means best adapted to maintain and prolong his life constitute the question to be solved. It has been said that "he who would long to be an old man must begin early to be one," but very few persons designedly take measures in early life in order that they may live longer than their fellows.

GROWTH, MATURITY AND DECLINE.

The whole term of life may be divided into the three main periods of growth and development, of maturity, and of decline. No hard and fast line can be drawn between these two latter phases of existence: the one should pass gradually into the other until the entire picture is changed. Diminished conservative power and the consequent triumph of disintegrating forces are the prominent features of the third period, which begins at different times in different individuals, its advent being mainly controlled by the general course of the preceding years. The "turning period," also known as the "climacteric" or "middle age," lies between 45 and 60; the period beyond may be considered as belonging to advanced life or old age. The majority of the changes characteristic of these last stages are easily recognisable. It is hardly necessary to mention the wrinkled skin, the furrowed face, the "crow's feet" beneath the eyes, the stooping gait, and the wasting of the frame. The senses, notably vision and hearing, become less acute; the power of digestion is lessened; the force of the heart is diminished; the lungs are less permeable; many of the air-cells lose their elasticity and merge into each other, so that there is less breathing-surface as well as less power. Simultaneously with these changes, the mind may present signs of enfeeblement; but in many instances its powers long remain in marked contrast with those of the body. One fact connected with advanced life is too often neglected. It should never be forgotten that while the "forces in use" at that period are easily exhausted, the "forces in reserve" are often so slight as to be unable to meet the smallest demand. In youth, the *vires in posse* are superabundant; in advanced life, they are reduced to a minimum, and in some instances are practically non-existent. The recognition of this difference is an all-important guide in laying down rules for conduct in old age.

In order to prolong life and at the same time to enjoy it, occupation of some kind is absolutely necessary; it is a great mistake to suppose that idleness is conducive to longevity. It is at all times better to wear out than to rust out, and the latter process is apt to be speedily accomplished. Every one must have met with individuals who, while fully occupied till sixty or even seventy years of age, remained hale and strong, but aged with marvellous rapidity after relinquishing work, a change in their mental condition becoming especially prominent. There is an obvious lesson to be learnt from such instances, but certain qualifications are necessary in order to apply it properly. With regard to mental activity, there is abundant evidence that the more the intellectual faculties are exercised the greater the probability of their lasting. They often become stronger after the vital force has passed its culminating point; and this retention of mental power is the true compensation for the decline in bodily strength. Did space permit, many illustrations could be adduced to show that the power of the mind can be preserved almost unimpaired to the most advanced age. Even memory, the failure of which is sometimes regarded as a necessary concomitant of old age, is not infrequently preserved almost up to the end of life. All persons of middle age should take special pains to keep the faculties and energies of the mind in a vigorous condition; they should not simply drift on in a haphazard fashion, but should seek and find pleasure in the attainment of definite objects. Even if the mind has not been especially cultivated, or received any decided bent, there is at the present day no lack of subjects on which it can be agreeably and profitably exercised. Many sciences which, twenty or thirty years ago, were accessible only to the few, and wore at best a somewhat uninviting garb, have been rendered not merely intelligible, but even attractive to the many; and in the domain of general literature the difficulty of making a choice among the host of allurements is the only ground for complaint. To increase the taste for these and kindred subjects is worth a considerable effort, if such be necessary; but the appetite will generally come with the eating. The possession of some reasonable hobby which can be cultivated indoors is a great advantage in old age, and there are many pursuits of this character besides those connected with literature and science. Talleyrand laid great stress on a knowledge of whist as indispensable to a happy old age, and doubtless to many old people that particular game affords not only recreation, but a pleasant exercise to the mind. It is, however, an unworthy substitute for higher objects, and should be regarded only as an amusement and not as an occupation.

Whatever be the sphere of mental activity, no kind of strain must be put upon the mind by a person who has reached sixty-five or seventy years. The feeling that mental power is less than it once was not infrequently stimulates a man to increased exertions which may provoke structural changes in the brain, and will certainly accelerate the progress of any that may exist in that organ. When a man finds that a great effort is required to accomplish any mental task that was once easy, he should desist from the attempt, and regulate his work according to his power. With this limitation, it may be taken for granted that the mental faculties will be far better preserved by their exercise than by their disuse.

Somewhat different advice must be given with regard to bodily exercises in their reference to longevity. Exercise is essential to the preservation of health; inactivity is a potent cause of wasting and degeneration. The vigour and equality of the circulation, the functions of the skin, and the aëration of the blood, are all promoted by muscular activity, which thus keeps up a proper balance and relation between the important organs of the body. In youth, the vigour of the system is often so great that if one organ be sluggish another part will make amends for the deficiency by acting vicariously, and without any consequent damage to itself. In old age, the tasks cannot be thus shifted from one organ to another; the work allotted to each sufficiently taxes its strength, and vicarious action cannot be performed without mischief. Hence the importance of maintaining, as far as possible, the equable action of all the bodily organs, so that the share of the vital processes assigned to each shall be properly accomplished. For this reason exercise is an important part of the conduct of life in old age; but discretion is absolutely necessary. An old man should discover by experience how much exercise he can take without exhausting his powers, and should be careful never to exceed the limit. Old persons are apt to forget that their staying powers are much less than they once were, and that, while a walk of two or three miles may prove easy and pleasurable, the addition of a return journey of similar length will seriously over-tax the strength. Above all things, sudden and rapid exertion should be scrupulously avoided by persons of advanced age. The machine which might go on working for years at a gentle pace often breaks down altogether when its movements are suddenly accelerated. These cautions may appear superfluous, but instances in which their disregard is followed by very serious consequences are by no means infrequent.

No fixed rule can be laid down as to the kind of exercise most suitable for advanced age. Much must depend upon individual circumstances and peculiarities; but walking in the open air should always be kept up and practised daily, except in unfavourable weather. Walking is a natural form of exercise, and subserves many important purposes: not a few old people owe the maintenance of their health and vigour to their daily "constitutional." Riding is an excellent form of exercise, but available only by a few; the habit, if acquired in early life, should be kept up as long as possible, subject to the caution already given as to violent exercise. Old persons of both sexes fond of gardening, and so situated that they may gratify their tastes, are much to be envied. "Fortunati nimium, sua si bona nôrint!" Body and mind are alike exercised by what Lord Bacon justly termed "the purest of human pleasures." Dr. Parkes goes so far as to say that light garden or agricultural work is a very good exercise for men past seventy: "it calls into play the muscles of the abdomen and back, which in old men are often but little used, and the work is so varied that no muscle is kept long in action." A few remarks must be made, in conclusion, with regard to a new form of exercise sometimes indulged in even by elderly men. I allude to so-called "bicycling" and "tricycling." Exhilarating and pleasant as it may be to glide over the ground with comparatively little effort, the exercise is fraught with danger for men who have passed the grand climacteric. The temptation to make a spurt must be often irresistible; hills must be encountered, some, perhaps, so smooth and gradual as to require no special exertion—none, at least, that is noticed in the triumph of surmounting them.

Now, if the heart and lungs be perfectly sound, such exercises may be practised for some time with *apparent* impunity; but if (as is very likely to be the case) these organs be not quite structurally perfect, even the slightest changes will, under such excitement, rapidly progress and lead to very serious results. Exercise unsuited to the state of the system will assuredly not tend to the prolongation of life.

With regard to food, we find from Dr. Humphry's Report that 90 per cent. of the aged persons were either "moderate" or "small" eaters, and such moderation is quite in accord with the teachings of physiology. In old age the changes in the bodily tissues gradually become less and less active, and less food is required to make up for the daily waste. The appetite and the power of digestion are correspondingly diminished; and although for the attainment of a great age a considerable amount of digestive power is absolutely necessary, its perfection, when exercised upon proper articles of diet, is the most important characteristic. Indulgence in the pleasures of the table is one of the common errors of advanced life, and is not infrequent in persons who, up to that period, were moderate or even small eaters. Luxuries in the way of food are apt to be regarded as rewards that have been fully earned by a life of labour, and may, therefore, be lawfully enjoyed. Hence arise many of the evils and troubles of old age, and notably indigestion and gouty symptoms in various forms, besides mental discomfort. No hard and fast rules can be laid down, but strict moderation should be the guiding maxim. The diet suitable for most aged persons is that which contains much nutritive material in a small bulk, and its quantity should be in proportion to the appetite and power of digestion. Animal food, well cooked, should be taken sparingly and not more often than twice a day, except under special circumstances. Dr. Parkes advocates rice as a partial substitute for meat when the latter is found to disagree with old persons. "Its starch grains are very digestible, and it supplies nitrogen in moderate amount, well fitted to the worn and slowly-repaired tissues of the aged." Its bulk, however, is sometimes a disadvantage; in small quantities it is a valuable addition to milk and to stewed fruits.

The amount of food taken should be divided between three or four meals at fairly regular intervals. A sense of fulness or oppression after eating ought not to be disregarded. It indicates that the food taken has been either too abundant or of improper quality. For many elderly people the most suitable time for the principal meal is between one and two P.M. As the day advances the digestive powers become less, and even a moderately substantial meal taken in the evening may seriously over-task them. Undigested food is a potent cause of disturbed sleep—an evil often very troublesome to old people, and one which ought to be carefully guarded against.

It is an easier task to lay down rules with regard to the use of alcoholic liquors by elderly people. A few years ago, the Collective Investigation Committee of the British Medical Association issued a Report on the Connection of Disease with Habits of Intemperance, and two at least of the conclusions arrived at are worth quoting. " Habitual indulgence in alcoholic liquors, beyond the most moderate amounts, has a distinct tendency to shorten life, the average shortening being roughly proportional to the degree of indulgence. Total abstinence and habitual temperance augment considerably the chance of death from old age or natural decay, without special pathological lesion." Subject, however, to a few exceptions, it is not advisable that a man sixty-five or seventy years of age, who has taken alcohol in moderation all his life, should suddenly become an abstainer. Old age cannot readily accommodate itself to changes of any kind, and to many old people a little good wine with their meals is a source of great comfort. To quote again from Ecclesiasticus, "Wine is as good as life to a man, if it be drunk moderately, for it was made to make men glad." Elderly persons, particularly at the close of the day, often find that their nervous energy is exhausted, and require a little stimulant to induce them to take a necessary supply of proper nourishment, and perhaps to aid the digestive powers to convert their food to a useful purpose. In the debility of old age, and especially when sleeplessness is accompanied by slow and imperfect digestion, a small quantity of a generous and potent wine, containing much ether, often does good service. Even a little beer improves digestion in some old people; others find that spirits, largely diluted, fulfil the same purpose. Individual peculiarities must be allowed for; the only general rule is that which prescribes strict moderation.

It is not to be inferred from the hints given in the preceding paragraphs that the preservation of health should be the predominant thought in the minds of elderly persons who desire that their lives should be prolonged. To be always guarding against disease, and to live in a state of constant fear and watchfulness, would make existence miserable and hasten the progress of decay. Selfish and undue solicitude with regard to health not only fails to attain its object, but is apt to induce that diseased condition of mind known as hypochondriasis, the victims of which are always a burden and a nuisance, if not to themselves, at least to all connected with them. Addison, in the *Spectator*, after describing the valetudinarian who constantly weighed himself and his food, and yet became sick and languishing, aptly remarks: " A continual anxiety for life vitiates all the relishes of it, and casts a gloom over the whole face of nature, as it is impossible that we should take delight in anything that we are every moment afraid of losing."

Sleep is closely connected with the question of diet: "good sleeping" was a noticeable feature in the large majority of Dr. Humphry's cases. Sound, refreshing sleep is of the utmost consequence to the health of the body, and no substitute can be found for it as a restorer of vital energy. Sleeplessness is, however, often a source of great trouble to elderly people, and one which is not easily relieved. Narcotic remedies are generally mischievous; their first effects may be pleasant, but the habit of depending upon them rapidly grows until they become indispensable. When this stage has been reached, the sufferer is in a far worse plight than before. In all cases, the endeavour should be made to discover whether the sleeplessness be due to any removable cause, such as indigestion, cold, want of exercise, and the like. In regard to sleeping in the daytime, there is something to be said both for and against that practice. A nap of "forty winks" in the afternoon enables many aged people to get through the rest of the day in comfort, whereas they feel tired and weak when deprived of this refreshment. If they rest well at night, there can be no objection to the afternoon nap; but if sleeplessness be complained of, the latter should be discontinued for a time. Most old people find that a reclining posture, with the feet and legs raised, is better than the horizontal position for the afternoon nap. Digestion proceeds with more ease than when the body is recumbent.

Warmth is very important for the aged; exposure to chills should be scrupulously avoided. Bronchitis is the malady most to be feared, and its attacks are very easily provoked. Many old people suffer from more or less cough during the winter months, and this symptom may recur year after year, and be almost unheeded. At last, perhaps a few minutes' exposure to a cold wind increases the irritation in the lungs, the cough becomes worse, and the difficulty of breathing increases until suffocation terminates in death. To obviate such risk, the skin should be carefully protected by warm flannel clothes, the out-door thermometer should be noticed, and winter garments should always be at hand. In cold weather the lungs should be protected by breathing through the nose as much as possible, and by wearing a light woollen or silken muffler over the mouth. The temperature of the sitting- and bed-rooms is another point which requires attention. Some old people pride themselves on never requiring a fire in their bedrooms. It is, however, a risky practice to exchange a temperature of 65° or 70° for one fifteen or twenty degrees lower. As a general rule, for persons sixty-five years of age and upwards, the temperature of the bedroom should not be below 60°, and when there are any symptoms of bronchitis, it should be raised from five to ten degrees higher.

Careful cleansing of the skin is the last point which needs to be mentioned in an article like the present. Attention to cleanliness is decidedly conducive to longevity, and we may congratulate ourselves on the general improvement in our habits in this respect. Frequent washing with warm water is very advantageous for old people, in whom the skin is only too apt to become hard and dry; and the benefit will be increased if the ablutions be succeeded by friction with coarse flannel or linen gloves, or with a flesh-brush. Every part of the skin should be thus washed and rubbed daily. The friction removes worn-out particles of the skin, and the exercise promotes warmth and excites perspiration. Too much attention can hardly be paid to the state of the skin: the comfort of the aged is greatly dependent upon the proper discharge of its functions.

Such, then, are the principal measures by which life may be prolonged and health maintained down to the closing scene. It remains to be seen whether, as a result of progress of knowledge and civilisation, life will ever be protracted beyond the limit assigned to it in a preceding paragraph. There is no doubt that the *average duration* of human life is capable of very great extension, and that the same causes which serve to prolong life materially contribute towards the happiness of mankind. The experience of the last few decades abundantly testifies to the marked improvement which has taken place in the public health. Statistics show that at the end of the septennial period, 1881—87, 400,000 persons were alive in England and Wales whose death would have taken place had the mortality been in the same proportion as during the previous decade. It may be reasonably expected that as time goes on there will be an increase in the proportion of centenarians to the population as a whole.

The question whether long life is, after all, desirable does not admit of any general answer. Much depends upon the previous history of the individual, and his bodily and mental condition. The last stages of a well-spent life may be the happiest; and while sources of enjoyment exist, and pain is absent, the shuffling-off of the mortal coil, though calmly expected, need not be wished for. The picture afforded by cheerful and mellow old age is a lesson to younger generations. Elderly people may, if they choose, become centres of improving and refining influence. On the other hand, old age cannot be regarded as a blessing when it is accompanied by profound decrepitude and disorder of mind and body. Senile dementia, or second childishness, is, of all conditions, perhaps the most miserable, though not so painful to the sufferer as to those who surround him. Its advent may be accelerated by ignorance and neglect, and almost assuredly retarded or prevented by such simple measures as have been suggested. No one who has had opportunities of studying old people can shut his eyes to the fact that many of the incapabilities of age may be prevented by attention to a few simple rules, the observance of which will not only prolong life and make it happier and more comfortable, but will reduce to a minimum the period of decrepitude. Old age may be an incurable disease, admitting of but one termination, but the manner of that end, and the condition which precedes it, are, though not altogether, certainly, to a very great extent, within our own power.

NOTE.—Since the above was written, the civilised world has lost its most noted centenarian in the person of M. Chevreul, the famous French chemist, who died on April 9th, 1889, aged 102 years and 7 months. Only a few days before his death he went in his carriage to see the Eiffel Tower, in which he took a lively interest. Throughout his long life he had worked hard, sparing neither mind nor body, and it would seem that his faculties were preserved with but slight impairment up to the time of his death. The senior member of the medical profession, Mr. W. Salmon, died May 10th, 1896, aged 106 years.

V.

CLOTHING AS A PROTECTION AGAINST COLD.

FOOD and raiment are primary necessaries of life, and the mutual relation between these requisites is so close that a deficiency of one may to some extent be compensated by a full supply of the other. When both are decidedly defective in quantity, marked symptoms soon become developed; exposure to cold intensifies the results of insufficiency of food. On the other hand, the effects of chronic starvation are mitigated and warded off for a time by the application of heat. The machinery of the human body must be kept at a certain temperature, the maintenance of which is provided for by the combustion of the materials of food. Clothing prevents the too rapid escape of the heat thus generated. If good cookery be the most important of arts, the second place may be fairly assigned to proper forms and methods of dress. I propose to submit a few considerations on clothing as a means of keeping the body warm, that is, of preventing undue loss of heat at times when the external temperature is far below that of the body.

Owing to the common use nowadays of the clinical thermometer, most persons are aware that the normal temperature of the human body is about 98·6° Fahr. It is, however, subject to important daily fluctuations, which have to be considered in estimating any decided alterations. It is sufficient here to notice that the human temperature falls to its lowest about one or two o'clock A.M., while the maximum daily temperature occurs some time in the afternoon. These variations are influenced by food; but as they occur in fasting persons, they are not altogether dependent upon the supply of nourishment. Exercise has a decided effect in raising the temperature, a fact of which every one is conscious. The application of cold, as by a cold bath, lowers the temperature of the skin, but raises temporarily that of the internal organs, as it causes an increased volume of blood to be forced into them. In hot countries the bodily temperature is raised, at all events in new-comers.

Perhaps the most wonderful phenomenon connected with the bodily temperature is the preservation of its general level under all external circumstances of heat and cold. This power seems to exist in man in a higher amount than in most other animals, since he can not only support but enjoy life under extremes which would be fatal to many. The accounts of degrees of cold frequently sustained by Arctic voyagers are almost incredible. We read of temperatures 80°, 90°, and even 102° below the freezing-point. On the other hand, in the tropics the temperature often rises through a large portion of the year to 110° or even higher, and we know that workmen can remain in furnaces at a temperature of 300° or more without inconvenience. In all these cases the air must be dry and still; similar extremes of heat or of cold accompanied by moisture would prove intolerable.

This power of spontaneous regulation of the temperature resides in a mechanism whereby more or less blood is sent to the skin as a result of relaxation or of contraction of its blood-vessels. When the skin is heated, its vessels relax and contain a surplus of blood, which, if exposed to ordinary external influences, rapidly becomes cooler. Heat is lost in three ways—viz., by radiation, conduction, and evaporation, the amounts given off by these means varying according to circumstances. It is estimated that about 70 per cent. of the whole amount of the animal heat passes off through the integument. If the skin be freely exposed to cool air, much heat is lost by radiation; if the air be dry and in motion, a still larger quantity of heat becomes latent by the evaporation of the water excreted by the sweat-glands. Thus it is that, under normal conditions, a rise in the bodily temperature causes a flow of blood to the skin, followed by cooling. A man warmed by exercise, and exposed to a current of air, rapidly becomes chilled, and perhaps catches cold. Lowering of the temperature, on the other hand, diminishes the quantity of blood in the skin, so that radiation and conduction of heat from the surface are reduced to a minimum. Evaporation and radiation from the internal surface of the lungs constitute another means whereby heat is lost; but for our present purpose it is unnecessary to do more than notice the fact.

The main use of clothing is to protect the body generally and to maintain it at an equable and proper temperature. Civilised man, who is compelled to wear artificial clothing, is so far less favourably situated than the lower animals, who are provided with sufficient natural covering. This drawback is, however, more than counterbalanced by the opportunities which clothing affords of rendering the wearer comparatively independent of external circumstances of climate.

The materials used for clothing are derived mainly from the animal and vegetable kingdoms. It is only necessary to mention the most important, and to refer to their properties.

From the animal kingdom we get wool, silk, furs, skins, leather, and feathers. The vegetable kingdom supplies us with cotton, flax, and their derivatives, and likewise with hemp, jute, indiarubber, gutta percha, etc. Wool is by far the most important article of clothing; it is a modification of hair, and is furnished by the sheep, goat, camel, and other animals;

wool consists of round fibres, made up of a number of little cornets which have become united. Under the microscope, the surface of the fibres is seen to present imbricated scales which all take one direction. These scales cause woollen fibres to adhere tightly together and make it difficult to unravel woollen cloths. Under the influence of moisture and pressure the interlacement becomes very close and firm, owing to the interlocking of the scales. The finest wools have the most numerous and pointed serrations; as many as 2,800 per inch have been counted in specimens of the finest Saxony wool. In old and worn wool these scales become indistinct, and are more or less obliterated. Besides forming cloth of various kinds, wool is made up into flannel, blankets, kerseymere, etc. Alpaca is the fleece of a genus of animals inhabiting South America; mohair is obtained from a particular kind of goat.

Shoddy is a modification of wool; its manufacture has developed into a large industry. It is made from old woollen cloth and woollen goods of all kinds; even old stockings, no longer worth darning, are convertible into shoddy. Having fulfilled their course, during which each article has perhaps clothed many different individuals, woollen materials of all kinds find their way to the shoddy-mill, in which they are torn asunder. After undergoing various processes of cleansing, the fibres are re-spun and re-woven with a certain admixture of fresh wool. If the original fabrics have been of good quality, the cloth containing the shoddy will present a very respectable appearance, but the wearing properties will be more or less impaired. The jagged serrations will have been worn away, and the fibres no longer cling to each other with the same degree of tenacity. After the shoddy-making process has been repeated several times, the fibres split up and become quite smooth.

Shoddy is now absolutely necessary for the clothing of mankind. If its manufacture were to cease, at least half our population would be deprived of woollen clothing. Even the best cloth may contain an appreciable amount of shoddy; the cheaper kinds may be almost entirely composed of it. Its presence is difficult to detect; the resisting power of cloth is the best means of determining whether shoddy has been mixed with new wool. Cloth ought to bear a certain weight before tearing, and at the Government Clothing establishments a machine is used by which the force required can be measured. Cloth containing shoddy is not only weaker and less resistant, but it is a less efficient protector against cold.

Silk is yielded by the silkworm, and consists of very fine tenacious filaments. It is the strongest of all textile materials, but unfortunately is capable of blending with many chemical substances in such proportions as to produce articles which may contain as little as 10 per cent. of true silk. Several salts of iron and tin, tannin, sumach, gambier, and other substances are capable of converting silk into expanded fibres, consisting of a conglomeration of more or less of these materials.

Fur has been used as an article of clothing from the earliest times. In Arctic countries it is, of course, indispensable. The combination of leather and hair is specially adapted to protect the body from wind and cold. Felt is made from the hair removed from the leather. The compactness and cohesiveness of felt are mainly due to the serrations already described as typical of hair.

Materials for clothing derived from the vegetable kingdom require only a short notice in this article. Of these, cotton is the most important; it consists of minute, exceedingly hard fibres, which absorb water slowly and scantily, and conduct heat much more rapidly than wool. As an article of clothing, linen closely resembles cotton, but it is a better conductor of heat, and absorbs water more freely.

The question as to the best material for clothing cannot be answered off-hand or in a few words. It has been urged that the "natural clothing" of animals is the "natural" and only proper clothing for the first of all animals—man. Dr. Poore thinks that an assertion of this kind is "in some degree similar to the old dogma that animal heat was different from other kinds of heat—a plausible theory, which the hatching of eggs in incubators by means of artificial heat has done much to explode."

The fact, however, remains that for certain purposes woollen clothing, furs, and skins cannot be replaced by any other materials. Experience teaches us that such is the case, and an explanation is not far to seek. In common language, certain fabrics are described as " warm," while others are classified as " cool." It is hardly necessary to say that neither warmth nor coldness is a property of the materials themselves. Some feel warm because they prevent the escape of the natural heat of the body—that is, they are bad conductors of heat; others feel cold, because they permit the bodily heat readily to pass off, and the cooler temperature of the air is no longer antagonised in the same degree. The source of the warmth is within the body, in like manner as the heat of a furnace is derived from the materials in process of combustion within it.

Now wool is a bad conductor of heat, and it owes much of its power in this respect to the amount of air entangled in the meshes formed by its fibres. The conducting power of linen and cotton is nearly twice that of wool. There is much probability in Dr. Poore's view that the power of different clothing materials in keeping the body warm depends more upon the amount of air entangled than upon the substances used in the construction of the fabric. Different materials are habitually woven in different ways, and "the fact that one material is warmer than another is often due to the fact that it lends itself by its nature to a particular mode of manufacture. Woollen materials are always more porous than linen fabrics, and it is mainly owing to this fact that the one is warmer than the other." Air, in common with gaseous bodies in general, is an extremely bad conductor of heat; but this property cannot be easily demonstrated, owing to the extreme mobility of particles of air. If such motion be hindered or retarded, the conductivity of air becomes very small. We make use of this property of air in various ways. If we wish to keep a liquid warm, it is placed in a vessel and surrounded by shavings, straw, and the like, which entangle large volumes of air in their meshes. A more obvious illustration is afforded by double windows, which are often used in cold climates to keep rooms warm. The effect is really due to the non-conducting layer of air interposed between them. It is for the same reason that two shirts are warmer than one of the same material, but of double the thickness. The Chinese and Japanese adopt the plan of wearing many layers of clothing, each layer being formed almost exactly like its fellow; by diminishing or increasing the number of layers, the wearers protect themselves against the vicissitudes of climate.

When the air is in active motion as well as cold, the necessity for non-conducting coverings is still more obvious. Wind carries off the layers of air in contact with the body, replaces them by colder air, and promotes evaporation whereby the temperature is lowered to an almost indefinite extent. Every one knows the sensation caused by wind blowing on damp clothes or on the wet skin, and the intense cold thus experienced. To obviate this effect, the wind must be prevented from reaching the surface of the body, and for this purpose skins and furs are the most efficient coverings. These constitute extremely warm clothing, and cannot be dispensed with in many parts of the world. It is perhaps well to repeat that these articles possess no warmth in themselves. When worn, they prevent the natural heat of the body from being rapidly dissipated and neutralised by the external cold air. Next to these come thick, coarse, woollen fabrics which entangle and retain large volumes of air. These are especially suitable whenever great fluctuations of temperature have to be encountered.

Besides the properties already mentioned, there is another peculiarity connected with wool which enhances its value as an article of clothing—viz., its power of absorbing water, which penetrates into the fibres themselves and causes them to swell, and also occupies the spaces between them. This property is a very important one as regards health. The normal skin gives off nearly a pint of water, in the form of perspiration, during twenty-four hours, and this fluid disappears by evaporation. The passage of liquid into vapour causes heat to become latent, and the bodily temperature is thus lowered, as may be clearly observed some little time after exertion. If dry woollen clothing be put on immediately after exercise, the vapour from the surface of the body is condensed in and upon the wool, and the heat which had become latent in the process of evaporation is again given off. Flannel clothes, therefore, put on during perspiration always feel warm, whereas cotton and linen articles allow the perspiration to pass through them, so that the evaporation and cooling processes are unchecked. There is, therefore, an obvious reason for selecting flannel clothing for wearing after active exertion. An individual who is perspiring freely is far less likely to take cold when clad in flannel than when clad in linen or cotton. Dr. Poore thinks that by adopting a looser method of weaving the material, cotton might be made to acquire properties similar to those of wool. If linen or cotton be woven "in a loose porous fashion, these fabrics then become, as heat-retainers, scarcely inferior to wool."

Woollen fabrics cause a sensation of warmth in virtue of another peculiarity which they possess. They often present a rough surface, which, coming into contact with the skin, causes friction, and therefore more or less warmth. The irritation thus produced is intolerable to some persons, but if it can be borne with for a short time the skin often gets accustomed to the sensation.

The colour of the materials has some influence on the warmth of clothing. Black and blue absorb heat freely from without, but white, and light shades of yellow, etc., are far less absorbent. This difference can be demonstrated by experiment; the same material, when dyed with different colours, will absorb different amounts of heat. In hot countries white coverings are universally worn, and sailors and others wear white clothing in hot weather. With regard, however, to heat given off from the body, the colour of the materials used as clothing makes little if any difference. Red flannel is popularly supposed to be warm, though it is no better in this respect than similar materials of equal substance but white or grey in colour. Dark clothing is best for cold weather, because it more freely absorbs any heat that is obtainable.

Waterproof clothing is very valuable under certain conditions. It protects against cold, rain, and wind; but it is an exceedingly hot dress, for it prevents evaporation, and condenses and retains the perspiration. Save for very short periods, it should never be worn by persons taking active exercise. For those, however, who are not exercising their limbs to any great extent, but are exposed to wet and cold, waterproof materials are an excellent protection. Woollen should be worn underneath in order to absorb perspiration, and the waterproof should be taken off as soon as the necessity for it has passed away. Ventilating waterproofs are sometimes offered; but a real combination of this kind is an impossibility. If a garment let out air and perspiration, it will let in wind and wet; if thoroughly waterproof, it will not admit of any true ventilation.

With regard to woollen clothing as a protection against wet, it must be remembered that fabrics of this kind, especially if loosely woven, absorb an enormous amount of water. A man clad in thick woollen clothes, and walking in rain for some hours without other protection, is conscious of great weight and inconvenience. Under similar conditions, cotton and linen garments are speedily saturated, and the wearer soon becomes chilled.

Garments made of pure silk are exceedingly comfortable, but very expensive. Thin silk, worn under flannel, adds greatly to the protection afforded by the latter against chills, and likewise prevents the unpleasant sensation of friction. Thin silken socks, worn under merino or woollen ones, form a good remedy for cold feet.

The principal conclusions to be drawn from the foregoing paragraphs may be thus briefly stated :—

1. As a protection against cold, woollen garments of equal thicknesses are much superior to either linen or cotton, and should always be worn for underclothing. Furs and leather are serviceable against great cold, and especially against severe wind. Waterproof clothing should be reserved for very wet weather, and generally for persons who are not taking exercise when exposed to it.

2. The value of several layers of clothing as compared with a single warm garment should be borne in mind. An extra layer even of thin material next the skin is often very valuable.

3. As a protector against cold, a garment should not fit closely to the body, but should be comparatively loose and easy, so that a layer of air is interposed between it and the

skin. A loosely woven material is warmer than one of an opposite character.

4. For wearing at night, woollen clothing is not generally desirable: cotton or linen is far better. The blankets constitute the woollen covering, and ought to protect the body sufficiently.

5. Lastly, it must always be remembered that the *source of heat* is *within the body* itself, and *not in the clothes.* Proper food coupled with a due amount of exercise will produce heat; the function of clothing is to retain the heat thus generated.

VI.

A CONTRIBUTION TO THE ALCOHOL QUESTION.

IN modern scientific treatises, articles taken as food are divided into two classes—food-stuffs and food-accessories. The first includes those animal, vegetable, and mineral products which are familiar to every one and are found necessary to life; the second, those beverages and condiments which have come to be regarded as essential to comfort. Controversy concerning the first class can scarcely be said to exist; the advocates of vegetarianism sometimes make themselves heard, but neither their precepts nor their examples are sufficient to overcome the force of habit and the dictates of common sense. The case, however, is far different with regard to one of the articles contained in the class of food-accessories. Certainly no subject of its kind has attracted more attention or given rise to more controversy.

The interest attaching to the use of alcoholic drinks is in great measure due to the terrible accumulation of evils, moral and physical, with which their abuse is associated. What mankind might have been in the absence of alcohol it is useless to speculate; the manifold changes which human beings undergo as a result of immoderate use are too easily discernible to require description. Too many of us can recall instances in which the ruin caused by alcohol entitles it to be called "the devil in solution."

There can be no difference of opinion as to the mental and physical degradation due to this agent, and to it alone; but, on the other hand, we are confronted with the very remarkable fact that the use of alcohol dates from very early times, and that it is well-nigh universal among civilised nations. It would appear, indeed, that the amount of alcohol consumed is proportionate to the degree of civilisation, and that, as regards capacity for work, the advantage is clearly with those races which use alcoholic drinks.

The widespread use of alcoholic drinks is due to the fact that their production is effected in the easiest possible manner, and that the requisite materials are to be found in most parts of the world. Given a solution of sugar, a ferment, and a due degree of heat, and alcohol is more or less rapidly formed. The sugar is broken up into carbon dioxide, most of which escapes in the form of gas, and alcohol, which remains in solution. The manufacture of alcoholic fluids is usually associated in our ideas with complicated apparatus, " plant," and large establishments; but these are requisite mainly because the products have to be supplied on a large scale, and in the form of palatable beverages. In the islands of the Indian Archipelago, and in many parts of Africa, an intoxicating drink is readily obtained by making incisions into a palm-tree, catching the juice in a suitable vessel, and allowing it to stand for a few hours.

Many questions are connected with the use of alcoholic drinks, and some of them justly excite the deepest interest, and for the following reasons: (1) the enormous consumption of such drinks in the United Kingdom and in other European countries; (2) the amount invested in their production and distribution; (3) their value, or otherwise, when taken in moderation; (4) the manifold evils, in the shape of poverty, crime, and disease, caused by excess. A consideration of the best means of inducing temperance or abstinence is invested with peculiar interest.

The effects of alcohol, in small, moderate, and large doses, have been minutely studied by a host of competent observers; and yet much difference of opinion exists as to the terms in which its general action may be accurately described. It is usually regarded as a stimulant; indeed, as the stimulant *par excellence*. On the other hand, in the opinion of some well-recognised authorities, the notion conveyed by the word "sedative" would best express the action of alcohol. In order to ascertain what ground there is for this latter view, it is necessary to refer to the effects of alcohol; they are conveniently divided into three stages, known respectively as excitement, intoxication, and coma or insensibility.

1. A small or moderate dose of alcohol (say two tablespoonfuls of brandy), properly diluted,

produces in an ordinary individual more or less distinct evidences of excitement. The heart beats more frequently and with more force, the superficial vessels are dilated, and hence the skin of the face and hands appears flushed, the eyes are animated and perhaps somewhat reddened, the intellectual faculties are excited, the individual is more disposed to joy and pleasure, cares disappear, and ideas flow with greater rapidity and ease. Under the influence of a somewhat larger dose, many persons exhibit a strong disposition to talk, very few are noticed to become taciturn; indiscretions of various kinds are apt to be committed. It has been often asserted that the true nature of the individual is brought out by alcohol; this question will be subsequently referred to. In any case, it is obvious that alcohol has a specific action upon the nervous system, the different parts of which it affects in a more or less definite order. It acts upon the nervous structures in a twofold manner: first, by coming into contact with them, and, secondly, by increasing and accelerating the circulation through them. Dr. Brunton thinks that the nervous tissues are affected in the inverse order of their development, the highest centres being affected first and the lowest last. Thus the power of judgment usually goes first, while the imagination may be lively and the emotions more than usually active; so that, after a man becomes incapable of discussion, he is combative, affectionate, or lachrymose. The motor centres may be next affected, either after or before the perceptive centres, so that the speech may be uncertain and thick while the power of judgment is little affected, or the speech may remain tolerably distinct after the power of clear conception is entirely gone. This condition, however, belongs rather to the second stage.

2. This is characterised by disorder of the intellectual functions and of the will, manifested by delirium and loss of power over voluntary muscles. To quote again from Dr. Brunton, the cerebellum appears to be affected sometimes before and sometimes after the cerebrum. This depends partly upon the constitution of the individual, and partly upon the quality of the alcoholic liquor. The affection of the cerebellum gives rise to double vision and inability to walk, from the relations of surround-

ing objects being no longer correctly perceived. After both cerebrum and cerebellum are paralysed, the spinal cord may still retain its functional activity, so that the man who cannot walk may be able to ride, owing to the reflex contraction of certain large muscles of the thigh produced by the impression of the saddle. This second degree is often accompanied by nausea and vomiting, a sense of exhaustion, and an irresistible desire for sleep, which may continue for some hours. When the person awakes, he is conscious of headache, thirst, malaise, loathing of food, and other disagreeable feelings. The varieties of the phenomena observed depend in the main upon the temperament of the individuals. A classification of drunkards can indeed be founded upon these peculiarities. Thus the surly, the melancholic, the nervous, the choleric, and the phlegmatic drunkard may be easily distinguished.

3. Coma or insensibility. This state, in which there is profound unconsciousness, is most often observed when large quantities of spirit have been swallowed in a short time. In many of its features it resembles apoplexy,

and mistakes are not infrequently made. Recovery is, of course, the rule; but death may ensue from paralysis of the heart or of the muscles of respiration.

The effects of the prolonged use of excessive quantities of alcohol, though differing in form in different individuals, are for the most part easily recognised. Digestion suffers; the appetites of drunkards are seldom normal; sickness and distaste for food are very common symptoms. The liver is very prone to become affected; the condition known as gin-drinker's liver has been recognised and studied from a very early period. It may doubtless be caused by other kinds of spirit; but the dram-drinker usually selects gin because of its low price, and hence the disease of the liver is called after the name of the particular spirit which generally occasions it. If alcohol be never taken in the neat state, but always freely diluted with water, there is far less chance of its causing this form of disease.

It is, however, in the nervous system that the effects of the chronic abuse of alcohol are most clearly marked. The tremulous hand, the quivering lips and tongue, and the unsteady walk are among the earliest signs. The will becomes weakened and the moral sense blunted; we meet with drunkards who are so completely the slaves of their tyrannical appetite for drink that they are ready to gratify it at any sacrifice. The explosions known as *delirium tremens*, which constitute a connecting link between intoxication and insanity, are due to poisoning of the blood and perverted nutrition of the brain; they are a measure of the degree in which the nervous system is implicated. But there are other results, less familiarly known perhaps, but of graver significance, and due to the implication of many of the large nervous trunks. These latter become inflamed, hardened, thickened, and painful, and there is loss of power in the limbs. This condition is more often seen in women than in men, and the lower extremities most frequently suffer. Complete paralysis is sometimes thus produced.

This sketch of the physiological action of alcohol would seem to prove that the effects of small doses are clearly of a stimulating character, but that these sooner or later pass off and are succeeded by others of an opposite kind. After large doses, the stage of excitement is very short, while the phenomena indicative of depression are apt to be very marked. The expression "dead-drunk" is not a whit too strong to describe the condition which alcohol is capable of producing. The total loss of motor power and the almost complete abolition of sensation closely resemble death. It is a well-known fact that drunken men often receive serious injuries without any consciousness of pain. But these sedative or anæsthetic effects of alcohol are made apparent in a very different manner, and are capable of being produced even by moderate doses. Dr. Wilks indeed asserts that it is really for the purpose of producing *sedative* effects that this so-called *stimulant* is eagerly swallowed by the multitude. He points to the fact that persons under the influence of grief not infrequently turn for comfort to alcoholic liquors, with the object of drowning their troubles in the bowl. It would be absurd for them to have taken a stimulant to excite greater manifestations of grief, or to make them feel their troubles more acutely. It would be easy to multiply examples of this kind, and to show that sedative effects are often sought for; but, on the other hand, alcoholic drinks are taken under precisely opposite conditions, and obviously for the purpose of stimulating feelings which are beginning to be experienced. Dr. Wilks' explanation will hardly account for the use of alcohol on these occasions. He maintains that its quieting effects constitute its great value at the dinner table. "Both Matthew Arnold and Wendell Holmes upheld its advantages in this respect. Without it, the guests would be quarrelling or keenly discussing political or religious subjects—with apologies to teetotallers—but wine comes in, rubs off the acerbities, and brings all down to the same level of good humour." It is surely more reasonable to suppose that wine in small quantities makes men more companionable by quickening the flow of ideas and by increasing temporarily the power of expression. Moreover, it creates a feeling of warmth and comfort, and excites the appetite.

In most discussions upon alcohol, and almost invariably among teetotallers, spirits, wines, and beer are placed in one and the same category, as if all were equally mischievous.

Common experience, however, shows that these liquors differ remarkably in their effects. If we compare wine with spirits, we find that the former possesses certain tonic properties not attributable to the latter. Again, the stimulating effect of wine is more slowly produced and lasts longer than that of spirits. But perhaps the most important distinction consists in the fact that the intoxicating influence of wine is less than that of a mixture, say of brandy and water, containing the same quantity of alcohol, and is not proportionate in different wines to the amount of alcohol they contain. Analysis shows that eight parts of brandy, by measure, contain about the same quantity of alcohol as eighteen-and-a-half parts of port wine. If the intoxicating power of various liquors were proportionate to the spirit contained in them, a pint of port wine would be almost equal to half-a-pint of brandy. We know, however, that such is not the case. Again, champagne contains less alcohol than claret, but is far more intoxicating. It would seem probable that the action of the alcohol is modified by that of the other constituents of the wine. As to the manner in which this effect is produced, it is impossible to speak with certainty. It may be that the other constituents are in chemical combination with the spirit, for it is generally admitted that a brandied wine—that is, a wine to which spirit has been *added*—is more intoxicating than a *natural wine* of the same alcoholic strength.

It is, of course, true that some of the most prominent effects of intoxicating liquors are directly due to the quantity of alcohol contained in each, though other ingredients must not be disregarded. Spirits contain about 50 per cent. of alcohol; wines vary greatly in this respect, the proportion in sherry and port sometimes rising as high as 25 per cent., while it may fall as low as 7 in Bordeaux and Rhine wines. Ordinary beer contains about 5 per cent., but in strong ales this proportion may be doubled. Besides alcohol, brandy contains minute quantities of various ethers. These are more numerous and abundant in wine, and give rise to the odours, in addition to modifying the effects of the alcohol. Beer contains, besides alcohol, a considerable quantity of sugar, with free acid and salts.

The differences between the effects of these

three classes of liquors are often clearly demonstrated in the cases of persons who take habitually immoderate quantities, but confine themselves for the most part to one form of liquor. Hogarth, in his well-known pictures, *Beer Alley* and *Gin Lane*, has faithfully represented the differences between topers devoted to malt liquor and dram-drinkers. He has depicted the former as rubicund, corpulent, and bloated; the latter, as pale, thin, or emaciated. Wine-bibbers are for the most part full-blooded and corpulent. The majority of drunkards, however, do not confine themselves to one class of liquors; though the practised dram-drinker usually despises all fluids less potent than spirits.

Much controversy has taken place on the important question as to whether alcohol undergoes any changes after being taken into the body, or whether it is eliminated unchanged. It is certainly absorbed by the mucous membrane of the stomach, and passes into the blood, by which it is conveyed to all parts of the body. At least a portion very soon begins to leave the tissues, for it can be detected in the breath shortly after it is taken, and smaller quantities escape by the skin and other organs. In cases of fatal intoxication, the odour of the alcoholic liquor can be detected in the fluid contained in the ventricles of the brain, and some authorities have supposed that a peculiar affinity exists between the brain-substance and alcohol. More recent investigations have shown that this fluid does not accumulate in any special manner in the nervous tissue. It has also been pretty clearly proved that alcohol, taken internally, is not entirely eliminated as such, but that some of it is decomposed in the system. As to the proportion thus changed, no exact statement can be made; but, admitting the fact, we cannot deny that alcohol is a *food* in the strict sense of the word. This inference is supported by those cases in which only minute quantities of ordinary aliment are taken during several months, or even years, but wines and spirits are freely administered, the patient meanwhile showing no loss of weight. Dram-drinkers, likewise, are often very small eaters. In both classes of cases the alcohol, besides acting as a food, doubtless checks waste and retards normal changes. It is sometimes found that persons losing weight on an insufficient diet not only regain the normal standard after a little alcohol has been added, but even go beyond it.

The effects of alcohol are often compared with those of opium, when taken to produce pleasurable excitement, sensations of comfort, or dreamy repose. In a general way, opium causes less change in the actions of the person indulging in it than is ordinarily observed after the use of alcohol. Its tendency is to act upon the moral feelings and sentiments, and to soften down excesses of all kinds, while the effect of alcohol is more commonly displayed in excitement of the lower propensities. De Quincey's own observations enabled him to estimate these differences with great accuracy and clearness. After asserting that no amount of opium could produce intoxication (though the spirit used to make the tincture might have that effect), he goes on to show that opium differs from alcohol not merely in the quantity of its effects, but in the quality. Wine disorders the mental faculties; opium introduces among them the most exquisite order, legislation, and harmony. Wine exalts the contempts and the admirations, the loves and the hatreds of the drinker; opium communicates serenity and equipoise to all the faculties, active or passive. It is most absurdly said of any man that he is disguised in liquor; for, on the contrary, most men are disguised by sobriety, and it is only when they are drinking that men display themselves in their true complexity of character, which is surely not disguising themselves. In short, the man who is inebriated, or tending to inebriation, is, and feels that he is, in a condition which calls up into supremacy the merely human, too often the brutal, part of his nature; but the opium-eater (if not suffering from any disease, or other remote effects of opium) feels, according to De Quincey, that the diviner part of his nature is paramount—that is, the moral affections are in a state of cloudless serenity.

In everyday life the practical questions with regard to alcohol are mainly two—viz., Is its regular use in small quantities a universal necessity? and are such small quantities mischievous, salutary, or practically without effect? It is around these questions that controversy is always raging, and occasionally assuming volcanic activity. Some years ago the columns of the leading journals were occupied for many weeks with letters on this subject. The impartial reader, after carefully perusing the various statements and opinions, many of them supported by facts of personal history, might say with Faust, *und bin so klug als wie zuvor*, or with Sir Roger de Coverley, that much might be said on both sides of the question.

Admitting, as we must, that alcohol is to some extent a food, we know that it is not taken for purposes of nutrition by the great mass of those who use it in moderate quantities. Persons who are honest and intelligent say that they take it because they like it; because it makes them feel more comfortable; because they enjoy their food better than when plain water is taken; because it helps them to sleep, etc. Now all these are perfectly valid reasons, and as such ought to be respected. They are not to be thrust aside by the assertion that such an auxiliary is a dangerous one, and that its good effects are much overrated, and, if not, are more than counterbalanced by others of an opposite character. Experience is unshaken by such assertions, and is strongly reinforced by the fact that alcohol, in some form or other, is in common use among civilised nations. It may well be asked, Is such experience to go for nothing?

It may be granted without demur that, to the healthy individual, alcohol is by no means a necessary article of diet. The same statement holds good of tea and coffee. Pleasant and useful as these beverages may be, they are not indispensable; their introduction was a great innovation, and their use was long confined to the wealthy. They are stimulants, producing a decided effect upon the nervous system; they are mischievous when taken in excess, and some people abstain from them altogether. Speaking broadly, they supply that craving for stimulants which seems to be innate in the human system; and, because they do this, their use has become so common.

No sweeping statement ought to be made as to the necessity for alcohol. In settling the question in any given case, we have to consider the surrounding physical conditions of the individual; his work, whether mental or bodily, whether hard or moderate; his food, whether plentiful and suitable, or the reverse. For a man in good health, well-fed, working with his limbs out of doors, alcohol is seldom, if ever, necessary, though it is often a very pleasant adjunct to one or more meals. A man who under such circumstances takes two or three glasses of beer daily is a temperate man, and ought to be regarded as such. I fully agree with Dr. Wilks that, in the class of society to which we belong, the beer-drinker is generally a temperate man; he seems content with his beverage, and to have no desire for anything stronger. No doubt many a man of this kind could get on almost, or quite, as well with water, but he prefers the beer, and therefore takes it. When great and sustained exertion is required, experience shows that alcohol is useless, if not mischievous. Soldiers endure fatigue and the extremes of heat and cold far better if alcohol be withheld. Dr. Parkes says that when debarred from spirits and fermented liquors, men are not only better behaved, but are far more cheerful, are less irritable, and endure better the hardships and perils of war. It is a well-known fact that drinking is the great source of all crime and insubordination in the Army, and that, although much improvement has been effected of late years, the belief is dominant in some quarters that ardent spirits impart strength and vigour to the human frame. The obstinacy with which men cling to this groundless belief would surprise those who attempted for the first time to combat this foolish prejudice.

For persons compelled to lead a sedentary life, a little alcohol taken with meals may be not only pleasant, but often extremely useful. It is found to help digestion, and to brace up and sustain flagging functions. In old age alcoholic stimulants are often very serviceable, especially in relieving sleeplessness, attended with slow and imperfect digestion. The late Dr. W. B. Carpenter, the most sensible and the most intelligent champion of the Temperance cause, found it desirable, in his old age, to take a little wine, and declared that he was the better for it. I purposely refrain from making any remarks on the use of alcohol in disease; this important topic is unfitted for discussion in these pages.

The greater longevity of total abstainers has naturally been used as an argument in favour of the practice, and it is one that deserves consideration, though it must not be pressed too far. To go to the other extreme, it is quite certain that the high rate of mortality among the intemperate is not sufficiently recognised. Dr. Ransome calculates that from 40,000 to 50,000 lives are lost every year from alcoholic indulgence. The numbers shown in the Registrar-General's reports fail to represent the actual mortality from this cause. Dr. Newsholme states that liver disease is perhaps the most trustworthy test of alcoholic excess, and that the mortality it causes is six times as high among innkeepers and publicans, and two and-a-half times as high among brewers as among the generality of males. In these classes the mortality from gout and nervous diseases is also invariably high, and alcohol likewise contributes to the mortality from phthisis.

The statistics of certain assurance offices apparently yield very striking evidence in favour of total abstinence as contrasted with moderation; but conclusions thus obtained are by no means absolutely to be relied upon. We never know what another person means by moderation unless we are fully acquainted with his habits of life and ideas on the subject. When we are able to ascertain the habits of so-called moderate drinkers, it often happens that the qualifying epithet is found to be quite out of place. Assurance offices refer to friends for the characters of applicants, who of course mention those who are likely to speak well of them. Their confidence is seldom misplaced; a free liver, taking himself as the standard, will return his friend as highly moderate or very temperate. Dr. Wilks quotes an American authority to the effect that insurance offices which admit moderate drinkers will always have a larger number of risks, and that from a third to one-half of all the inebriates under his care have life policies. It is obviously unfair to compare total abstainers with a class containing so many drunkards. Companies who admit moderate drinkers, and leave the question of risk in these cases to the judgment of examiners, will always have a large number of these dangerous risks and a larger mortality. " What we want is a comparison between total abstainers and really moderate drinkers. We have this in the tables published by the United Kingdom Temperance Association and the Clergy Mutual Assurance. Among the clergy we have abstainers and moderate drinkers, but very few intemperate lives, so that we may well compare them with the total abstainer." Dr. Wilks states that, so far as he can understand the tables, the clergy, including the moderate men, have a slight advantage over the total abstainers. We have no statistics enabling a comparison to be made between the lives of spirit-drinkers and those of wine-drinkers. Even if pure examples of both types were procurable in sufficient numbers, it would be impossible to eliminate the influence of other agencies favourable or unfavourable to longevity. It must also be borne in mind that there are at least two classes of total abstainers: those who have never tasted the accursed thing, and those who have become abstainers because at some time or other of their lives they have tasted a great deal too much of it. Even if other conditions were equal, the prospects of longevity for individuals belonging to these two classes would necessarily be very different. There is another point, already alluded to: we have no right to attribute a definite effect to one cause alone when other probable causes exist. Abstinence from intoxicating drinks may well indicate a man's general character, other features of which will be favourable to longevity. Total abstainers may be credited with the possession of superior prudence in other matters. Long-lived persons are often early risers; but it is more probable that the vigorous vitality maintains the habit than that the habit alone maintains the vitality.

To return to the question of moderation in the use of alcohol, although different persons have very different ideas on this subject, certain experiments made by the late Dr. Parkes and others have enabled a satisfactory and definite conclusion to be drawn. In a strong, healthy man accustomed to alcohol in moderation, the quantity given in twenty-four hours that begins to produce effects which can be considered injurious is something between one and two fluid ounces. If this quantity be exceeded, certain effects indicate the advent of that stage in the greater degrees of which the poisonous effects of alcohol become manifest to all. The experiments were made upon two powerful, healthy men, and the conclusions therefore apply to such alone; in women, the quantity required to produce decidedly bad effects would in all probability be less. For children (except as a medicine in illness), alcohol is always mischievous, and the very small quantity which suffices to produce intoxication in them indicates that they absorb it rapidly and tolerate it badly.

The quantity of alcohol above mentioned must be regarded as the maximum; but as it is expressed in absolute spirit, it is necessary to ascertain how much it represents of ordinary spirituous liquors. Dr. Parkes tells us that one ounce is equal to two ounces of brandy (or whisky), to five ounces of the strong wines (ports, sherries, etc,), to ten ounces of the weaker wines, or to twenty ounces of beer. If these quantities are increased by one-half (corresponding to one and a half ounces of absolute alcohol), the extreme limit of moderation for strong men will be reached. Any additional quantity must be deemed excessive and certainly injurious.

As supplementing Dr. Parkes' estimate, much interest attaches to some experiments made by Sir W. Roberts on the effects of alcoholic fluids on the various stages of the process of digestion. It appears that spirits, in dietetic quantities, have no influence on salivary digestion, but wines, probably by virtue of their acidity, check the activity of this process. Gastric digestion is unaffected in the presence of 10 per cent. of proof spirit; but 20 per cent. retards operations, and 50 per cent. altogether checks them. The retarding effect of wine and malt liquors is not proportionate to the amount of alcohol contained in them; something else is present which has a more decided effect in this direction. Sherry and port have the most retarding effect; half a pint of sherry at dinner would make a mixture in the stomach containing 25 per cent. of the wine. This proportion would check digestion, and could only be deleterious. Malt liquors have a less retarding effect, but the latter becomes noticeable when 20, 40, or 60 per cent. of these fluids are added.

The fact that alcohol in somewhat full doses

tends to retard digestion raises the question as to whether such retardation can ever prove beneficial. If this question can be answered in the affirmative, do we obtain a reason why alcoholic liquors are so frequently taken with meals? Sir W. Roberts thinks it quite possible that digestive retardation is sometimes useful, and that men take alcoholic beverages in part with the unconscious purpose of compassing this result. At first sight, it appears strange that great pains should be taken in cooking to make our food digestible and easy of attack by the digestive fluids, and that we should swallow liquids which render such culinary efforts more or less nugatory. Dr. Roberts explains the incongruity on the ground that if the food be rendered too easy of digestion, there arises a risk that the meal will pass too quickly and wastefully into the blood, and on through the tissues into the excretory organs, and so out of the body, before it has been made fully and economically available for the sustenance of the slow nutritive processes. Moreover, a sudden irruption into the blood of large quantities of newly digested aliment would tend to disturb the chemical equilibrium of that fluid, and so interfere with the tranquil performance of its functions. It would also tend to produce congestion of the liver and other organs, to the general disadvantage and discomfort of the economy. A too rapid digestion and absorption of food may be compared to feeding a fire with straw, instead of with slower burning coal. In the former case, it would be necessary to feed often and often, and the process would be wasteful of the fuel; for the short-lived blaze would carry most of the heat up the chimney. To burn fuel economically, fires are often damped down in order to ensure slow as well as complete combustion. The same process may often be advantageously applied in the digestion of food. There is nothing contradictory in making nutritive materials as digestible as possible, and controlling the rate of digestion by the use of certain accessory articles with food. This explanation refers to ordinary eating and drinking; but it also throws light on the adage that "Good eating requires good drinking." Immoderate meals are sometimes ended by slow soaking in dilute alcohol of almost all the food taken. Digestion is thus checked and prolonged, and in extreme cases the abdominal canal gets rid of its contents after a very scanty absorption of their nutritious principles into the blood-vessels. Some of the direct consequences of gourmandising are thus obviated.

I have now alluded to the principal points connected with the use of alcoholic liquors by persons in health. It would be easy to refer to other branches of the subject; but to do so at any length would transgress the limits of an ordinary article. I would observe, in passing, that the Duchess of Rutland's remarks in the *New Review* (Jan. 1892) on the best methods of combating intemperance are well worthy of perusal, and very encouraging to all workers in this field, Those who are anxious to know what steps the German Emperor proposed to take in order to combat intemperance will find their wants supplied by Mr. Beatty Kingston's interesting pamphlet on the subject as a whole, Much doubtless remains to be done, but the progress made during the last few decades justifies the brightest hopes for the future. The state of opinion in most circles with regard to drunkenness is a striking indication of the progress made, but by no means the only one. Some portion of this improvement is due to the teetotallers, but deductions must be made for the consequences of the intemperate language of many advocates of the latter class. The evils of intemperance can scarcely be exaggerated, but to fling strong epithets at those who are really temperate only provokes a reaction in favour of drink. In the early days of the teetotal movement it was the habit to show far more abhorrence for moderate drinkers than for actual drunkards. The latter were represented as victims, the former as seducers, the drunkard being tempted into guilt by the example of the moderate. Fanatical declamation was the rule, and hence it came to pass that a teetotaller was commonly regarded as either a knave or a fool. Had it not been for the well-known eminence and honesty of men like the late Dr. Carpenter, the teetotal cause might have been crushed by the weight of ridicule evoked by those who claimed to be its champions.

All this is changed now; there are, of course,

a few fanatics, some of whom, unfortunately, while always clamouring for the help of legislation, too often prevent any good from being achieved by its means. In the opinion of the author, little, if any, improvement can be expected from legislation; the precepts and examples of the temperate will continue to operate, though without the noise and fuss so dear to the fanatical and ignorant. Let us regard alcohol as a luxury for most of those who take it, as a necessity for some persons, and as a poison for others; let us educate children to do without it; let us deal with habitual drunkards as we do with lunatics; let there be continuity in our views and actions, and let us be very careful not to substitute intemperance of thought and word for intemperance in alcohol.

VII.

FASTING AND ITS PHYSIOLOGY.

ATTEMPTS to discover the period during which a human being can exist without food, in the ordinary sense of the term, have often been made, and have excited an amount of interest out of all proportion to their scientific value. There is reason to believe that, as might have been expected, serious damage to health was the sole result of the experiment in all cases, and that such damage was but poorly compensated by the pecuniary reward which was the usual cause of the experiment. It is certain that the inducement in some form or other must be enormous to cause a sane man to endure such great and prolonged suffering.

The human body in some respects resembles a steam-engine; it performs work and requires fuel in the shape of food, which, when converted into tissue, furnishes the motor power, the quantity of food required varying with the work done. We may assume that a ploughman requires more food than a tailor, just as a locomotive burns more fuel than a small engine. When very little work of any kind is done, a very little food goes a long way; if food be withheld altogether, the machine does not stop, for the body itself can be used to supply the fuel, without the necessity for immediate restoration by means of food. The body, therefore, differs from an engine in one very essential point; the latter cannot consume as fuel the materials of which it is composed, but all its power is derived from the coal or coke in the furnace, and is in direct proportion to the amount consumed. When the supply of fuel is exhausted, the machine stops. The animal organism, on the contrary, consumes its own body; it burns its tissues, and not its food; but the latter is required to make good the loss. Long after the food has been transformed into the solids and liquids of the living body, the animal organism can go on working and manifesting all its ordinary powers. There is, however, a limit to this consumption of the tissues; the man who takes no food resembles a spendthrift who lives upon his capital—when the latter is exhausted, the end comes. Meanwhile, in the case of the fasting man, the gradual destruction of his tissues is attended by very marked changes.

The symptoms of fasting have been very carefully studied by means of experiments upon animals, and the information thus obtained has enabled us better to comprehend the phenomena displayed by human beings when deprived of food. The following were the principal symptoms noticed by M. Chossat, a French investigator:—The animals remain calm during the first half or two-thirds of the period; they then become more or less agitated, and this state continues so long as their temperature remains fairly high. Some hours before death the temperature rapidly falls, and the animal becomes still, and remains in any position in which it is placed. As the coldness becomes more marked, the weakness increases, the breathing becomes slower, and insensibility gradually passes into death. One important fact must not be overlooked, inasmuch as it illustrates the risks to which Succi and others exposed themselves. Chossat found that sudden death was not uncommon in starving animals long before the ordinary time, and that the slightest shock was sufficient to destroy life at once. A pigeon kept fasting for a long time falls down and dies when its claws are clipped; whereas it would have lived for several days if not interfered with. This sudden death occurs from what is termed "syncope"—the heart's action is at once arrested when a sensitive nerve is painfully excited. A very slight smart of pain is quite sufficient to cause immediate death in animals thus reduced to a condition of great debility. There is no reason why the same accident should not occur in the human subject, and if "a fasting man" were thus suddenly to expire, it would be a matter of remorse for those who encouraged him in his attempt.

The loss of weight in fasting animals was carefully determined by Chossat, and he found that it amounted on the average to 40 per cent., but there was a considerable difference between the extremes, and this seemed to depend upon the amount of fat previously accumulated in the body, those animals in which the fat had been most abundant losing the most weight, but living the longest. The above-mentioned proportion may, however, be exceeded, and the animal may yet survive. Some years ago a fat pig was buried in its sty for 160 days under 30ft. of the chalk of a cliff at Dover; it was dug out alive at the end of that time, reduced in weight from 160lb. to 40lb., or no less than 75 per cent.

The most remarkable facts connected with the loss of weight are that the fat is almost completely used up, no less than 93 per cent. being removed; the heart loses 44, the muscles in general 42, the bones 17, while the nervous system loses barely 2 per cent. It is evident, therefore, that death occurs when the stock of combustible material is consumed, and that every other tissue gives up its components so as to save the nervous system as much as possible.

The immediate cause of death from fasting is, in reality, the reduction of the bodily temperature, which must ensue when all the available combustible material is used up. At first the fall is very gradual, but afterwards the decline is more rapid until the reduction amounts to nearly 30 degrees below the normal point, and death then takes place. Chossat noticed that if whilst in the state of torpor preceding death the animal was artificially warmed and its temperature raised, some amount of consciousness and muscular power was gradually restored, and if food were then cautiously administered, some of the animals experimented upon escaped from impending death. Young animals kept without food died sooner than older ones, and, contrary to what we should expect, no very decided difference was made in the duration of life either by withdrawing or permitting the supply of water.

The possible duration of life, when all food, save water, is abstained from, is the question which experiments like those, for example, of Dr. Tanner and Succi have at least partially solved. Admitting the reality of the former's fast, it would follow that life can be sustained for forty days on water alone. There are, however, other cases which show that this period may be considerably exceeded. In 1831 a murderer at Toulouse, in order to escape public execution, committed suicide by abstaining from food for sixty-three days. At first, efforts were made to feed him by force, but his violence was so great that these were abandoned, and only ineffectual persuasion was resorted to. During the sixty-three days, he consumed between eight and ten pints of water, on some days taking only a few drops. In the case of the Corsican prisoner, Viterbi, who committed suicide by starvation, life was prolonged for twenty-five days only. It is stated that he took a little water from time to time. Some years ago the notorious poisoner, William Palmer, when under sentence of death in Stafford Gaol, refused food for several days, in the hope of cheating the hangman. On being told, however, that he would be forcibly fed if he persisted in this course, he at once abandoned it.

Cases of voluntary abstinence for long periods are not unfrequently met with in medical practice. In one, recorded a few years ago, a lady, aged sixty, much distressed by some family trouble, suddenly refused food. She adhered to her determination, and died on the forty-ninth or fiftieth day, having taken nothing but cold water, with the exception of two teaspoonfuls of brandy on one occasion. There were no grounds for suspecting any deception. In another case, also that of a lady, aged eighty, life was prolonged for thirty-three days under conditions of total abstinence from food, a few spoonfuls of water daily excepted. The authenticity of the fast was perfectly assured; she kept quiet in bed, talked but little, and took little notice of those about her. At the end of the first week delirium came on, but ceased after a few days. There was no craving for food, and, inasmuch as there was no physical exertion, the wear and tear of the tissues was reduced to a minimum.

The case of the Welsh fasting girl, Sarah Jacobs, which excited a painful interest twenty-seven years ago, was of a very different character. The girl was an impostor, and, aided by her parents and others, had pretended to abstain from food for many weeks, but had not lost flesh. In order to clear up the mystery, she was placed under systematic inspection, and she died eight days afterwards from acute starvation. During the greater part of this time she was cheerful, and exhibited nothing extraordinary. Later on it was found that she could not be kept warm, and she gradually sank into a torpid state, which continued till death. It was a terrible experiment, and one which was utterly unjustifiable. The girl, who was only twelve-and-a-half years old, should have been taken from her friends and treated in a hospital. There was no emaciation visible after death, and, indeed, more than the average amount of fat was present. The rapidity with which death ensued was due to the want of water.

Seventeen years have elapsed since Dr. Tanner's prolonged fast, which was begun in New York, June 28th, 1880. He was an eccentric man, of respectable character and strong self-will, who endeavoured to make amends for an assumedly unsuccessful medical career by promulgating various startling theories on the subjects of electricity and fasting. During the first nine days, he swallowed only a quarter of a pint of water, which, however, he used freely to rinse his mouth and bathe his feet. He found, however, that further abstinence from fluid was impossible; on the eleventh day he began to take water freely, swallowing about five quarts during the next four days, and gaining in bodily weight about 4½lb. It was only natural that this change should excite considerable doubt as to the reality of his fast. He used to go out daily, taking rides and drives, but spent most of his time curled up in his bed. He was reported to be in very poor condition three days before the expiration of the term; but he accomplished his task, and, according to his own account, without pain or severe distress. He was never delirious. His experiment was unfavourably regarded by the orthodox physicians of New York, and they declined to witness it. He therefore placed himself under the care of the so-called "eclectics," who undertook the task of watching him. One remarkable feature connected with his fast was that he did not attempt to husband his resources by reducing the action of his lungs and heart to a minimum.

There is no doubt that some of the conditions under which Dr. Tanner was placed were decidedly unfavourable, and there are various circumstances which must exert a modifying influence, and either increase or diminish the period during which life can be sustained in the absence of food. Other things being equal, a stout person has a chance of living longer than a thin one, inasmuch as he possesses a larger store of combustible material which will serve him as fuel. Exposure to cold in conjunction with starvation always accelerates death, while a moderately high temperature aids in prolonging life. The presence of moisture in the atmosphere has a similarly favourable effect, inasmuch as it diminishes the exhalation of fluid from the body. It is probably owing to warmth and moisture that persons buried in mines or confined in some similar manner have had their lives preserved beyond the ordinary period. Dr. Tanner's success was, no doubt, favoured by the summer heat of New York. In the case of some miners, four men and a boy, who were imprisoned in a portion of a mine for eight days without food, but within reach of water, all were rescued alive and well. The warmth and dampness of the compressed air were, doubtless, favourable circumstances. In another case, recorded by Foderé, some workmen were extricated alive after fourteen days' confinement in a damp vault, in which they had been buried under a ruin. Dr. Sloan has given an account of a still more remarkable instance, in which a healthy man, aged sixty-five, was found alive after having been shut up in a coal-mine for twenty-three days, during the first ten of which he was able to get at a little water. He was, however, much exhausted, and died three days afterwards, although very carefully treated. In morbid states of the nervous system, life may be prolonged in the most extraordinary manner in the absence of food. In a remarkable case, recorded by Dr. Willan, of a young gentleman who starved himself under the influence of a religious delusion, life was prolonged for sixty days, during the whole of which time nothing but a little orange juice was taken.

Somewhat analogous to the cases just mentioned are those in which all food is abstained from while the person is in a state of trance or partially suspended animation. This state may be prolonged for many days or even for weeks, provided that the body be kept sufficiently warm. The most remarkable instances of this character have been furnished by certain Indian fakirs, who are able to reduce themselves to a state resembling profound collapse, in which all vital operations are brought almost to a standstill. In one case, the man was buried in an underground cell for six weeks, and carefully watched; in another, the man was buried for ten days in a grave lined with masonry, and covered with large slabs of stone. When the bodies were disinterred, they resembled corpses, and no pulsation could be detected at the heart or in the arteries. Vitality was restored by warmth and friction. It is probable that the fakirs, before submitting to the ordeal, stupified themselves with bhang (Indian hemp), the effects of which would last for some time, and the warmth of the atmosphere and soil would prevent any serious loss of heat, such as would soon occur in a colder climate, when the processes by which it is generated are made to cease.

The most prominent symptoms of starvation, as noticed in the human subject, are due first, to the special sensations produced by the absence of food and fluid, and, secondly, to the decline in the physical and mental powers. At first there is great uneasiness or severe pain in the region of the stomach; this is relieved by pressure, and subsides after a day or two, but is followed by a feeling of weakness and sinking in the same region, accompanied by intolerable thirst, which, if water be withheld, becomes the chief source of distress. The skin over the whole body is withered or shrivelled, and has lost its elasticity; the countenance becomes pale and cadaverous; the sufferer has a wild look; he loses flesh and strength more or less rapidly; he totters in walking, and becomes less and less capable of exertion. The mental power likewise fails; at first there is usually a state of torpidity, which may advance to imbecility; in some cases delirium comes on before death, in others the patient is attacked by convulsions, which speedily bring the scene to a close. After death the state of the body, as regards wasting, resembles that of animals: the fat has almost entirely disappeared, the blood is reduced to three-fourths of its normal amount, and the muscles are extensively wasted; the brain and nerves alone have suffered slight decrease in weight. If a little water has been procurable, the quantity of blood may be comparatively normal, though the quality is seriously changed.

If we compare this general description with that presented by Signor Succi after three parts of his fast had been completed, it may appear not a little exaggerated. Succi was pale, thin, and wasted, but the change was nothing like so great as one would expect. Many a patient, convalescent from typhoid fever, has an aspect of greater emaciation and weakness, and certainly could not write a few words with the same degree of firmness. The temperature of Succi's apartment was decidedly high, and the air charged with moisture, both of which conditions are favourable. He appeared to take no exercise beyond that involved in passing from his bed to his chair, and in sitting up for several hours daily. Besides water (pure and mineral), of which he took about a pint daily, he swallowed a few drops of a so-called "elixir," the composition of which was kept a secret. If it did not contain morphine, its effects were probably similar to those of that drug. It was said to allay pain and discomfort in the stomach.

Various tests were adopted in order to measure the changes that took place in Succi's bodily system, as the result of his prolonged fast. The loss of weight is, of course, easily ascertained. At the beginning of the experiment, Succi's weight was about 126¼lb. His decrease in thirty days amounted to 28lb. 13oz., or just 2oz. more than he lost during his last fast, of thirty days, at Brussels. A loss beyond one-fourth of the bodily weight is scarcely compatible with life, but this limit may be reached. He had not, however, the advantage of a large proportion of fat when he began his fast. It has been estimated that a very fat man has about 33lb. of fat at his disposal, and that this quantity would last him for fifty days. Dr. Tanner, during his fast, is said to have lost 32lb. only. In a prolonged fast, such as we are now considering, the daily loss becomes comparatively very slight during the last three weeks. Succi, for instance, on the thirtieth day, lost only 6oz., whereas under normal circumstances, a healthy adult loses 2lb. of solid matters daily.

Besides losing flesh, a fasting man loses to some extent the power of generating heat, and his temperature therefore falls. The normal temperature of the body is about $98\frac{1}{2}°$, and its source is the food taken into the stomach and the oxygen of the air absorbed by the lungs during respiration. Succi's temperature on the thirtieth day, for example, was about two degrees below the normal, a difference not to be wondered at when we remember that he lost only 6 oz. in weight in the twenty-four hours, and that all his disposable stock of fat had probably been consumed. Small as the loss may appear to be, the accompanying temperature, if discovered in a sick person, would be regarded as that of collapse; and if the thermometer marked only 95°, there would certainly be extreme danger.

A marked proof of the diminution in bulk is afforded by the instrument called the spirometer, which enables us to measure the capacity of the lungs. This latter, in Succi's case, if we again take the thirtieth day, was reported to be 1,450 cubic centimetres, or 88 cubic inches. These numbers represent the volume of air expelled from the chest by the deepest expiration following the deepest inspiration. The instrument itself consists of a tube, furnished at one end with a mouthpiece, and at the other connected with a gasometer of registered and graduated capacity, into which the person breathes. Now, in health, an adult 5ft. 8in. in height, after taking a deep breath, can expel from his chest about 238 cubic inches of air. Succi's chest capacity was at first 2,000 cubic centimetres, and it had, therefore, been much reduced; but a portion of the difference was doubtless due to the lessening of his muscular power.

Succi's loss of strength, as shown by the dynamometer, was comparatively small. This instrument consists of a ring of steel, to the inner face of which is attached a brass semi-circular dial, graduated with two rows of figures representing pounds or kilogrammes. When the steel ring is compressed by the hand, its short diameter is lessened and, by means of rack-work, an index moves to and fro on the scale. The power of the muscles of the hand and arm vary with the strength of the person experimented upon, and the dynamometer enables us accurately to ascertain the variations. It must be admitted that persons using the dynamometer daily, become more expert in concentrating their strength upon the spring, and a little allowance must be made on this account. Succi's amount of strength, as recorded by the dynamometer, was somewhat exaggerated, but when all allowance is made for increased expertness, the change was very small indeed.

VIII.

THE SPREAD OF DIPHTHERIA.

IN the autumn of 1894 the daily newspapers contained an appeal, of a somewhat novel character, from Sir Joseph Lister, as Chairman of the Council of the British Institute of Preventive Medicine. He stated that a new and highly successful method of treating a terrible disease, rapidly increasing in frequency, and in its severe forms almost or altogether intractable, had recently been discovered. The marvellous potency of the remedy had been demonstrated by a host of cases in which the gravest symptoms had disappeared under its application; and certain additional advantages were claimed for it—namely, that the treatment was perfectly harmless, and that it was prophylactic as well as curative in its effects. Such a concurrence of advantages has seldom, if ever, been paralleled, and it is not to be wondered at that the preparation of the remedy involved processes of the utmost delicacy, and was therefore somewhat costly, and that the supply fell short of the demand. The disease referred to is known nowadays as *diphtheria*—a name only too familiar in many households; and the new remedy has been termed *antitoxin*. Sir Joseph Lister appealed for funds to enable the Institute over which he presides at once to take in hand the preparation of *antitoxin* on a large scale. It was fitting that one who has already done so much to prevent disease and to save life should place himself in the foreground of the battle against diphtheria.

Before adverting to this new treatment and to the steps which led to its discovery, it seems desirable to give a brief sketch of the history of the complaint, and to notice the circumstances which tend to promote its spread. On this latter topic a large amount of evidence has accumulated during the last few years, but some portions of the subject are still involved in obscurity.

In 1856 a serious disease of the throat began to be very prevalent in this country. Many deaths occurred, and much alarm was naturally created. It was generally regarded as a new phenomenon; for many distinguished physicians, including Dr. Addison and Sir T. Watson, confessed that they had never met with similar cases. Dr. Watson, indeed, averred that while practising in London for more than twenty-five years, he had scarcely so much as heard of such a disease. Before any outbreak actually occurred in this country, reports had become common that a disease of the throat was causing great mortality at Boulogne. When cases appeared at home, the symptoms were found to be identical with those noticed on the other side of the Channel, and the epidemic was therefore stigmatised as the "Boulogne sore throat."

It is a very common practice, among individuals and communities, to impute misfortunes of all kinds to the agency of others, or at least to external sources, and the history of medicine furnishes several examples of this propensity. The more serious the epidemic, the greater the proneness to seek for its origin in some other country. In the case, however, of this particular outbreak, there was ample justification for applying to the malady, at least provisionally, the name of the place whence it spread to this country. The epidemic broke out in Boulogne early in 1855, and lasted until March 1857. The disease was especially common and severe among the English residents—a somewhat numerous contingent at that time. It caused 366 deaths, 341 of which were among children under ten years of age. Scattered cases began to appear in England in 1855, and in the following year many towns and districts experienced severe visitations. From that time the complaint has seldom been absent from this country, and in recent years there has been a very considerable increase in the number of cases.

" The term " diphtheria," or rather " diphtherite," was first applied to the disease, in 1821, by M. Bretonneau, a physician at Tours. It is derived from a Greek word signifying a prepared hide or piece of leather; and the disease was so named because of its essential feature—viz., the presence of a layer of more or less tough membrane in various parts of the throat. Bretonneau was fully aware of the fact that diphtheria was by no means a new disease. He considered that the outbreaks observed by himself were identical in character with some epidemics described by certain Italian and Spanish physicians of the seventeenth century. There is, moreover, good reason for believing that the disease prevailed in very early times. Aretæus, a Greek physician of Cappadocia, who flourished about 100 A.D., has left a description of a disease which corresponds in all particulars with diphtheria as seen at the present time. He tells us that Egypt and Syria engender the complaint, which thence derived the name of Egyptian and Syrian ulcers.

In the records of epidemics down to the end of the sixteenth century, there are many statements which would seem to apply to outbreaks of diphtheria. But the first absolutely reliable information about the complaint dates from the end of the sixteenth and beginning of the seventeenth centuries. It comes from Spain, where the disease continued to prevail for more than thirty years. The Spaniards called it Garottillo, which was originally the name applied to the small truncheon used in Spain by the executioner to strangle criminals. A few years later the complaint broke out in

Naples, and afterwards in Sicily, where it caused great mortality among children.

About a hundred years elapsed before the disease again became prevalent in an epidemic form. In 1739 a very severe affection of the throat was observed in London, and some seven years later it caused great mortality at Bromley in Middlesex, and at Greenwich. A very minute and clear description of the disease and its symptoms was given by Dr. J. Fothergill in 1748. Not long afterwards epidemics occurred near the Metropolis, and in various towns and villages in Devonshire and Cornwall. In some of these outbreaks scarlet fever and diphtheria were intermingled, as sometimes happens at the present day. Birmingham was subsequently visited. At Chesham, in Bucks, it was especially noticed that the complaint was not confined to the town, which lies in a valley, but appeared likewise with equal violence upon the neighbouring hills at a distance of five or six miles. Various parts of Europe experienced similar visitations at this period; and about the middle of the century the disease extended to America.

Thenceforward the spread of the disease

can be definitely traced. Bretonneau's *Memoirs* contain the earliest account of any epidemic during the present century, though Dr. Mackenzie, of Glasgow, had noticed isolated cases as early as 1812. The epidemic of Boulogne sore throat in 1855 marks an epoch in the history of diphtheria. There is every ground for hope that 1894 will be known as the year in which the disease was first successfully combated.

As already stated, the essential characteristic of the disease is the presence of a membranous layer or coating, ash-grey in colour, in various parts of the throat, and sometimes in the nose. But before this appears, or at any rate before it is detected, there is generally more or less headache, weakness, difficulty of swallowing, pain in the throat, and fever. The symptoms are, therefore, both local and general ; and they are liable to present great differences in their intensity and duration. No case, however mild its symptoms, is altogether free from danger. In some forms the patients recover in a few days, never having felt really ill; in others, after a very serious condition has existed for perhaps a fortnight, improvement sets in and a favourable termination ensues.

On the other hand, death may occur two or three days after the first appearance of the symptoms, or may follow at a later period, as a result of one or more of the many complications which are wont to occur. Between the mildest and the most severe cases innumerable gradations exist. The average mortality varies in different epidemics; it generally ranges between 25 and 40 per cent. During the last few years the number of fatal cases has been steadily increasing in London, though the proportion of deaths to attacks has considerably diminished. In the metropolitan area in 1889, the deaths from diphtheria numbered 1,617; in 1892, they were 1,969; while in 1893, they reached a total of 3,265. During the second quarter of the year 1894, 644 deaths were registered from diphtheria, and 1,826 from the same cause in England and Wales. Recent observations, extending over eight years, in Prussia, show a yearly average mortality of more than 40,000 children from diphtheria, the number of deaths almost equalling the fatality from scarlet fever, measles, and whooping-cough combined.

The fact that the mortality from diphtheria

has more than doubled in London during the twenty years terminated by 1890, and has, moreover, increased to a less extent throughout England and Wales, and especially in many cities and towns, cannot fail to excite alarm, not unmixed with surprise. During this period many sanitary laws have been passed, and their provisions have been vigorously carried out by a numerous staff of well-trained and competent officers. The public, as a body, is decidedly in favour of sanitary measures, and, for the most part, welcomes with avidity any arrangements likely to prevent disease. The beneficial effects of sanitary measures adopted in recent years have been often demonstrated; deaths from such diseases as scarlet fever and typhoid, which respond directly to sanitation, have undergone a substantial reduction during the period under consideration, while the case with regard to diphtheria is of a very different character. It is surely worth while to endeavour to account for this remarkable difference.

Inasmuch as the spread of diphtheria appears to be unchecked by sanitary measures, some authorities have gone so far as to assert that the disease is in the main independent of sanitary conditions or hygienic circumstances; but this view is nowadays not generally held. It is true that diphtheria sometimes prevails where the sanitary arrangements appear to be excellent, and fails to invade places of an entirely opposite character. The inference would seem to be obvious; but it is safer to assume that insanitary surroundings of all kinds tend to favour the spread of the disease, perhaps directly, but certainly by lowering the general health and the capacity for resisting infection. In the opinion of many medical officers of health, the existence of surface ventilators from the main sewers in the neighbourhood of houses is a possible, and even probable, cause of the spread of diphtheria. In Bristol the sewers have no external means of ventilation through grids and shafts, and the road gullies, after being water-trapped, are carried direct to the sewers. The death-rate from diphtheria is very low, and a similar experience is reported from Woolwich, where there are no surface ventilators connected with the sewers. This question assuredly demands further investigation.

The extraordinary spread of the disease in recent years is probably owing to a variety of causes. Increased means of communication must have exercised a more or less decided influence; but there are other factors of a still more potent character. It has been frequently observed, during marked epidemics, that certain localities were far more prone to be visited than others, and that such places were among the first to be attacked in subsequent outbreaks. These localities may be regarded as offering specially favourable conditions for the growth and development of the poison introduced from without; or, according to another theory, the germs of the disease may have lain dormant during the non-epidemic period and reacquired their activity on the return of favourable conditions of an unknown character.

Season and climate exert but little influence on the development and spread of diphtheria, but the disease is more common in temperate and cold climates than in the tropics. European statistics show that, in many epidemics, the maximum of sickness has occurred in the colder months, and the minimum in the warmer. There are, however, many exceptions to this statement.

Opinions differ as to whether varieties of soil exercise any influence in the development and spread of diphtheria. Dr. Hirsch states that the disease has been as prevalent in elevated as in low-lying places, in mountainous regions as on the level ground, on plains as in valleys, on dry as on wet soil, on the most varied geological formations, on porous and hard rock equally. But recent observers attribute more or less importance to dampness of soil in the production and spread of diphtheria.

It has been already observed that children are far more liable than adults to be attacked by the disease, and the liability is greatest between the ages of three and twelve. The mortality is greater during the first five years of life than at any other period. It is greater among females than among males; and this difference, which increases with the age of the children, is in great measure due to the larger share taken by girls in attending to household duties and in waiting upon the sick.

As the result of countless experiments and observations, it may now be regarded as certain that the symptoms of diphtheria are due to the action of a specific micro-organism, which was discovered by Löffler. Hosts of other organisms are found in the false membrane or coating; but little, if any, importance can be attached to them, inasmuch as germs of many kinds find an appropriate soil in dead tissues exposed to the air, and even in the mouth itself. It is now claimed that a distinct bacillus, which, when inoculated upon certain animals produces diphtheria, has been isolated and cultivated with success. These organisms have the power of producing a chemical poison in the diphtheritic membrane of the throat, whence it is absorbed by the system.

Long before the word "bacillus" was coined, observers were agreed as to the eminently contagious character of the malady. The occurrence of several cases in the same house, or in the same street, might, of course, be due to the fact that all the sufferers had been exposed to a common cause; but many instances are on record proving beyond the possibility of doubt that the disease may be distributed from the sick to those about them. In not a few cases medical men have fallen victims to diphtheria, after receiving in the nose or mouth a fragment of membrane coughed up by a patient. Such actual and visible contact with the virus is, however, not necessary, for the poison, in an invisible form, may pass through the air. Moreover, it would seem to cling with great tenacity to clothes and bed-linen, and even to the walls, woodwork, and furniture of rooms in which cases have been treated. Dr. Squire states that in a country house in Scotland, a visitor was attacked by the disease after occupying a room in which a case had occurred eleven months previously. It is probable that the virus can be carried only for short distances by currents of air, for in many epidemics cases are restricted to a few houses or to a single street, and the surrounding neighbourhood escapes.

It is highly probable that the spread of diphtheria is promoted in a very special manner by the massing together of large numbers of children, as occurs at the present day in many of our elementary schools. This view has been forcibly advocated by Dr. Thorne, who has paid great attention to the subject. He points out (1) That school attendance brings together those members of the community who are, by reason of age, most susceptible of diphtheria. (2) The children thus brought together are placed, and remain for many hours of the day, in exceptionally close relation with each other. Transmission of the virus is facilitated by the closeness of the mouth of the affected person to the mouth of the recipient, while the collective singing among the children and the consequent forced expiratory efforts must tend to diffuse the exhalations far and wide. (3) The closer the aggregation, and the more defective the ventilation, the greater the risk. (4) Any faulty sanitary surroundings render the children especially liable to receive infection in the presence of any case of diphtheria. (5) There are ample grounds for believing that the aggregation of children in elementary schools constitutes one of the conditions under which a form of disease of particular potency for spread and for death may be, so to speak, manufactured. (6) The danger of school aggregation is by no means limited to the period in which the disease is acute. (7) The practice of kissing and of transferring sweetmeats from mouth to mouth, as also the joint use of drinking-cups, etc., must be credited with a share in the diffusion of diphtheria. The fact must always be borne in mind that in not a few cases the disease assumes a very mild form. There may be no appreciable fever, and the general health is little if at all disturbed. Many children retain their appetites, and would, if left to themselves, run about the house as usual. Such cases are especially dangerous to the community, for the nature of the complaint may not at first be suspected. Meanwhile, other children become infected, and may soon present all the symptoms of a terribly severe attack.

But besides dissemination by contact and through the medium of the atmosphere, other channels of propagation have been discovered during the last few years. Milk may absorb the virus from patients, and communicate the disease to those who drink it. But a still more singular fact has been brought to light in connection with milk as a medium of propagation—namely, that epidemics have occurred in which the poison was derived, not from a human source, but from the cows themselves. Dr. Klein has shown that these animals can be successfully inoculated with cultures of the diphtheria bacillus, with the result that an eruptive disease is produced on the teats and udders. A few days after the inoculation, the presence of the diphtheria bacillus could with certainty be demonstrated in the milk of the cow, collected under all precautions. Dr. Klein justly remarks that these results lead in great measure to a right understanding of certain epidemics of milk-diphtheria. It is worthy of note that in cows the poison does not affect the organs of the throat.

Evidence is likewise at hand of the occurrence of diphtheria, sometimes with severe changes in the throat, among other domestic animals—for example, cats, horses, sheep, and fowls. The popular idea that a cat with symptoms of a cold in the head is a source of danger to children may hold good with regard to a much more dangerous disease. In houses containing patients suffering from diphtheria, cats have been known to present certain peculiar symptoms, "either antecedently, coincidently, or subsequently, they appear to have some kind of throat illness and cannot swallow; they sneeze, and their eyes water; bronchial mischief is noticed early, and the animals often become emaciated, and many die." Although the throat remains free from diphtheritic membrane, peculiar and striking changes are found in many organs of the body. A similar disease exists naturally among cats, and is believed to be equivalent to human diphtheria. Dr. Klein, therefore, considers that the cat is susceptible of diphtheria, and capable of communicating the disease to other cats and also to human beings.

Enough has been said to show that diphtheria can be propagated through various channels, and to account, in some degree, for the increase in the number of cases during recent years. It remains to consider the measures calculated to check the prevalence of the disease and to describe the remedy lately introduced.

The notification and isolation of cases ought,

of course, to be sedulously carried out; but there are several difficulties in the way. Sore throat is a very common complaint; it is, indeed, one of the symptoms of an ordinary cold, and a condition which may pass into diphtheria may exist for many hours without exciting the least suspicion. When cases of diphtheria occur in any locality, all forms of throat disease ought to be carefully investigated and examined by a medical practitioner. The efficient ventilation of schools would do much to check the spread of all infective diseases. If natural ventilation could not be achieved, artificial means of supplying fresh air ought to be adopted, notwithstanding the expense of any such method. When a case of undoubted diphtheria has occurred among children attending a school, the buildings should be forthwith closed and thoroughly disinfected. As a matter of course, the sufferers should be isolated, and visits from other children should be strictly forbidden. The milk-supply will require special attention, and all insanitary conditions should be remedied as far as possible. The object of sanitarians, however, is to prevent the occurrence of infectious diseases

—a task confessedly difficult, though not impossible. It is, however, a sad mistake to leave things alone until an epidemic occurs; yet even at the present day this practice is not very uncommon. In a parish not far from London, and containing some 1,700 inhabitants, we read that from the spring of 1893 up to February 1894 there were 77 cases of diphtheria, with 19 deaths. The conditions are thus described: The dwellings are fair, the sewerage *nil*, the drainage nuisances many, and the existing water-supply dangerous in the extreme.

With regard to the treatment of diphtheria, it is sufficient to say that remedies almost innumerable have been proposed and tried, and, in many cases, with apparent success. There are, however, forms of diphtheria practically hopeless from the very first. Treatment both local and general, is, of course, adopted, but the progress is always from bad to worse. The rate of mortality sufficiently indicates the impotence of medicine. Under such circumstances, the discovery of a method by which very severe forms of the disease may often be successfully combated must be hailed with intense satisfaction. The remedy, now called *antitoxin*, is the serum or watery part of the blood of animals rendered immune by repeated inoculations. This fluid is analogous to the attenuated vaccine virus of small-pox obtained from a child inoculated with the product of the virus of small-pox passed through the cow.

The method of preparing antitoxin is as follows:—The animals which are to furnish the antitoxic serum are rendered immune by the subcutaneous injection of the toxin of diphtheria. This toxin is formed when the virulent bacillus is grown in broth: after three or four weeks, the culture is sufficiently rich in toxin to be used. The animals employed are horses in good health, previously shown to be free from glanders. The culture, filtered through a porcelain filter, yields a clear liquid, with which the horse is inoculated by injection under the skin. Gradually, by repeated injections extending over two or three months, the horse is brought into a condition in which its serum possesses very high antitoxic properties. The animal does not suffer in health at all, or only to a very slight degree. The efficacy of its serum having been ascertained by a test experiment on a guinea-pig, the animal is bled. It suffers little from this operation, which may be repeated, if necessary, in a few weeks. "The animals used are cab horses, sound in constitution, but broken down in limb, who after inoculation live a life of ease and luxury, varied by a periodical phlebotomy, such as our grandfathers submitted to voluntarily two or three times a year."

The credit attaching to the discovery of *antitoxin* has been claimed, by many ill-informed Parisian newspapers, for a French physician, M. Roux. As a matter of fact, however, the microbe of diphtheria, *antitoxin* and its application, were discovered by German physicians, whose experiments and observations have simply been repeated by M. Roux and others. According to the *British Medical Journal*, M. Roux himself states that Löffler and Klebs discovered the microbe of diphtheria and studied its life-history; Roux and Yersin demonstrated that the bacillus was capable of evolving toxic material, and Behring crowned the edifice by discovering the antidote.

Since the introduction of the *antitoxin* treatment, many reports have been received as to its effects in a large number of cases occurring in our own country, in Australia, Germany, France, Austria, and the United States. The mortality, as compared with that of cases treated in other ways, shows a very remarkable decrease, the percentage of fatal cases having been reduced by one half or more. In no instance has a careful comparison of the statistics been unfavourable to the *antitoxin* treatment. This difference cannot be explained by supposing that the cases treated were of an unusually mild character. Among 520 cases at the Trousseau Hospital, Paris, where the treatment was not employed, the mortality was equal to 60 per cent. During the same period, in the Paris Children's Hospital, the mortality was less than 24 per cent., among 448 children treated with *antitoxin*. Similar and even more striking results have been obtained in Germany. In 1895 the Ministry for Medical Affairs instituted an investigation into the effects of *antitoxin*. The table of statistics included 6,626 patients of all ages, suffering from diphtheria. Of these, 86·5 per cent. recovered; 12·9 per cent. died, the remainder (less than 1 per cent.) being still under treatment. I may mention that my friend, Surgeon-Major General Paterson, late Principal Medical Officer at Aldershot, informed me that the treatment had been employed in about 400 cases in that station, and with marvellous results.

Enough has been adduced to show that in *antitoxin* we possess the most efficient remedy that has ever been used in the treatment of diphtheria. There is, moreover, good ground for believing that the injection of antitoxic serum enables the organism to resist subsequent infection with the microbes of diphtheria. It is satisfactory to know that arrangements have been perfected to ensure the supply of this valuable remedy.

IX.

THE PROPAGATION AND PREVENTION OF CHOLERA.

THE belief at one time prevailed that epidemic cholera appeared for the first time in India in 1817. The truth is that in that year the disease raged with terrible severity in the Delta of the Ganges; but it had already on several occasions desolated these regions. In 1781 cholera attacked a force, about five thousand strong, marching through Southern India; seven hundred died within the first few days, and some three hundred invalids were left behind. Two years later, cholera broke out at the sacred bathing spot at Hurdwar, on the Ganges. It happened to be one of the twelfth years deemed particularly propitious by the Hindoos, and the assemblage of pilgrims was far beyond the common average, amounting, it was said, to nearly two millions. The disease broke out on the springing up of an easterly wind during the night, and carried off innumerable persons. Twenty thousand victims are said to have fallen in less than eight days, yet so confined was its influence that the disease did not extend beyond the place of bathing and ceased on the dispersion of the multitude. The reports of the Medical Boards of Bengal, Madras, and Bombay contain accounts of similar epidemics in 1787, 1790, and 1814.

But the writings of the older physicians render it more than probable that the disease in an epidemic form was not unknown to our forefathers in Europe, and many of the cases described by Sydenham in 1669 would appear to have been true cholera. Inasmuch, however, as none of the visitations described by former writers approached in duration, severity, and extent that which took its rise in Bengal in 1817, no detailed record of them has been preserved. It is not to be wondered at that so terrible a visitation should have almost obliterated the memory of former outbreaks. Starting from its home on the banks of the Ganges, the pestilence invaded the districts and countries traversed by the Indus, Euphrates, Nile, Danube, Volga, St. Lawrence, and Mississippi. It visited almost every nation of the earth, unchecked by vicissitudes of climate and peculiarities of soil, circumscribed or limited by no prevailing wind; and whether it attacked the delicate frame of the Hindoo or the more robust European, the nature of the disease has been essentially the same, and the results of medical treatment have been for the most part unsatisfactory. Everywhere throughout the four quarters of the globe, experience has shown that no difference of race, climate, or temperature has exercised any marked influence on the nature and progress of the disease.

Various conditions of life, however, as in most other epidemics, have manifested their vast influences for good or evil: as shown amongst the poorer classes by their greater liability to this terrible scourge, and among the wealthier and more comfortably situated classes by their comparative exemption.

One fact of great importance is that the cholera epidemics which have ravaged various parts of India since 1817, and have spread therefrom to other countries, have always originated in India. They have never been even supposed to have been imported into any of the ports of India by ships from infected countries, or through any other manner of human intercourse. It may therefore be inferred that the cause of the disease, however latent or submerged for a time, is never actually absent from the soil of India in some of its parts.

Travelling, then, from place to place, in defiance of all natural and artificial barriers, under opposite extremes of temperature, season, and climate, against adverse winds, over lofty mountainous chains, across wide seas, passing (as Milton describes Satan) through "heat, cold, moist, and dry," how, one may naturally ask, is this terrible disease propagated?

As Sir T. Watson points out, the first thought that occurs to one's mind is that man also, and man alone, so far as we can perceive, overcomes all these kinds of hindrances to his locomotion, and therefore that the exciting cause of cholera in all probability accompanies and depends upon the movements of human beings over the earth.

If we inquire into the views held at various times with regard to the manner in which cholera spreads, we shall find that many differences of opinion have prevailed; but that at the present day there is a much nearer approach to unanimity. Not very long ago the complaint was pretty generally attributed to some poison present in the air; it was thought to progress by a succession of local outbreaks, the particular localities being chosen by certain local conditions: first, those which render places insalubrious; and, secondly, peculiar susceptibility to the disease on the part of the inhabitants of the place.

A second theory referred the disease to a morbid poison, which undergoes increase only within the human body, and is propagated to the healthy by means of emanations from the sick—*i.e.*, by contagion.

The third theory, propounded by the late Dr. Snow, and therefore deserving of special notice, gives a more specific form to the doctrine of contagion. It supposes that the poison of cholera is swallowed, and acts directly on the mucous membrane of the intestines, is at the same time reproduced in the intestinal canal, and passes out, much increased, with the discharges; that these latter afterwards, in various ways, but chiefly by becoming mixed with the drinking-water in rivers and wells, reach the alimentary canals of other persons and produce the like disease in them. This third theory is now generally accepted, as accounting in great measure, if not entirely, for the epidemic spread of cholera. There are, however, some instances on record for which this theory does not afford a sufficient explanation, and which seem to require a belief in some other modes of propagation. It will be well to take a brief survey of the evidence in favour of the transmission of cholera through the medium of drinking water.

Prior to 1849 very few of those who had opportunities of investigating cholera appear to have imagined that the specific poison might gain access to the human body in this way. Occasionally, as by Dr. Jameson in the Bengal Report of 1820, and by Dr. Müller, of Hanover, in 1848, hints were thrown out, but only in a cursory way, as to the effect of impure water in the production of cholera.

A decided addition was, however, made to our knowledge in 1849. In that year a severe epidemic of cholera prevailed in London, and carried off 6 per 1,000 of the population. The water used at that time was obtained in part from the rivers Thames and Lea, and in part from shallow wells. Sewers had been constructed, and closets, which drained into them, were in common use. Hence the river-water had become decidedly more impure than in 1832, the date of the previous epidemic, in which the mortality was a little over 3 per 1,000. In 1849 it was observed that the population supplied with water from the Thames suffered in direct proportion from cholera according as the water consumed was taken from the river at successively lower points. Thus, of those supplied with water taken from the river at Kew, 0·8 per 1,000 died of cholera; among those supplied with water drawn at Hammersmith, the mortality was 1·7 per 1,000; in the West of London, the water being taken at Chelsea, 4·7 per 1,000 died; while of those farther East and supplied with water taken between Battersea and Waterloo Bridge, the mortality from cholera was as high as 16·3 per 1,000 of the population.

If we search the records of a subsequent visitation of cholera in the year 1854, we shall find that a similar rule prevailed, with certain curious features which only pointed to the same conclusion as regards the part played by the water. In 1854 the river Thames was in all probability much more impure than in 1849, yet the Southwark Water Company still drew its supply from the river at Battersea, not far from the outlet of one of the sewers. In Bermondsey, which was supplied with water by this company, the deaths from cholera were 13 per cent. higher than in 1849, an excessive difference in proportion to the increase of population. In the interval between 1849 and 1854 the Lambeth Water Company had gone much farther up the river for a supply of water, viz., to a point above the tidal lock at Teddington. It so happened that in certain streets the pipes of the Lambeth and of the Southwark Water Companies interlaced, so that adjacent houses were supplied with water from different sources. On comparing the mortality, it was found that in the houses supplied by the latter company with water drawn from Battersea the deaths from cholera were 57·1 per 1,000 residences, whilst in those supplied from the Thames above London and the tidal influence, the mortality was only at the rate of 11·3 per 1,000 houses. Sir J. Simon, commenting on these facts, justly termed them as amounting to a gigantic crucial experiment performed on half-a-million of people. The history of another outbreak at the East End of London, in 1866, distinctly pointed to the drinking water as the medium of propagation. The outbreak occurred in a certain district which was "almost exactly the area of a particular water supply, nearly, if not absolutely, filling it, and scarcely, if at all, reaching beyond it."

The lesson to be drawn from another epidemic would appear to be quite conclusive. In 1854 there was a very remarkable local outbreak of cholera in the neighbourhood of Golden Square, Soho. It was investigated with great care and minuteness by a committee appointed for the purpose, and their report contains the most convincing evidence that the poison of cholera, in that instance at any rate, found its way into the body through the water used for drinking. The facts are briefly as follows:—During August 1854 there were a few cases of cholera in the locality; on September 1st the disease became very prevalent and very fatal, and the cases went on increasing in number during the four subsequent days. The complaint then began to abate. During the month of September 609 persons (14.2 per 1,000) fell victims to the epidemic, which was remarkable for the suddenness of its outbreak and the large number of persons simultaneously attacked. It was found on investigation that in the centre of this district there was a certain pump connected with a well, and that the radius of the infected area measured less than three hundred yards from the source of supply. The water of this well was much liked by the people who used it; it was cool, sparkling with carbonic acid gas, and kept well, owing to the quantity of saline matter it contained. On examination it was discovered that the water was contaminated by leakage and filtration from a cesspool at the time of the cholera outbreak, so that the possibility of the cholera poison gaining access to the water was fully demonstrated. Dr. Snow proved that the outbreak, properly so called, was in great measure confined to the neighbourhood of the pump, and that the water had been habitually used by sixty-one out of seventy-three persons who died during the first two days. In a factory, where the water was daily drunk, 9 per cent. of those employed died from the disease. On the other hand, in the workhouse, where the water supply was drawn from other sources, the deaths from cholera were only one-tenth of the proportion prevalent in the neighbourhood. Moreover, in a brewery in the very street that contained the pump, there was not a single case among the seventy men employed, who did not make use of the water.

If further proof were wanting of the communicability of cholera through drinking water, it is furnished with all the force, if not with the reality, of an experiment, by the facts thus stated by Mr. Macnamara, an Indian surgeon of great experience: "I may mention the circumstances of a case in which the most positive evidence exists as to the fact of fresh cholera dejections having found their way into a vessel of drinking water, the mixture being exposed to the heat of the sun during the day. Early the following morning, a small quantity of this water was swallowed by nineteen persons. (When partaken of, the liquid attracted no attention either by its appearance, taste, or smell.) They all remained perfectly well during the day; ate, drank, went to bed and slept as usual. One of them, on waking next morning, was seized with cholera; the remainder of the party passed through the second day perfectly well, but two more of them were attacked with cholera the next morning; all the others continued in good health till sunrise on the third day, when two more cases of cholera occurred. This was the last of the disease; the other fourteen men escaped absolutely free from diarrhœa, cholera, or the slightest malaise."

This account contains several points of great interest. In the first place, the choleraic dejections did not touch the soil; they were swallowed as passed, but after copious dilution with four or five gallons of impure water, and the mixture had been exposed to the light and heat of a tropical sun for twelve hours. It is also important to observe that in one case the poison produced its effects in twenty-four hours, and in the others, not until two or three days had elapsed. Lastly, it was evident that the majority of those who drank the polluted water escaped unhurt, an experience which proves that some persons are much more liable than others to take the complaint. A similar rule is often observed in connection with the spread of other infectious diseases. There is still much difference of opinion as to whether the poison of cholera floats about in the air, and is wafted by the winds and carried for considerable distances. The tendency of modern experience is, however, strongly against the theory of air-conduction. Mr. Macnamara only goes so far as to say that in badly ventilated rooms the atmosphere may become so fully charged with the exhalations from patients suffering from cholera as to poison persons employed in nursing the sick. In the same way, people engaged in carrying the dead bodies of those who have died from cholera, or in washing their soiled linen, may contract the malady. He adds that " in a dried condition, the poison contained in cholera excreta may retain its dangerous properties for a long time." This last statement is, however, at variance with the opinions of recent observers.

The not unfrequent outbreak of cholera among the crews of ships after they have been at sea for several days has been thought to prove the communicability of the disease through the medium of the atmosphere. Dr. Bryson, however, in a report published some years ago, stated that the medical records of the naval service had been searched in vain to discover an instance in which either cholera or yellow fever had made its appearance among a ship's company unless one or more of the men or officers had previously—within at most twenty-one days—been exposed in some house, ship, or locality where the infectious virus which emanates from persons ill of the one or the other of these diseases existed. The spontaneous origin of either malady, far away from an infected locality, is unknown in the naval service.

In connection with the above statement, the account of an outbreak of cholera on board the emigrant steamer *Dorunda*, in 1885, possesses considerable interest. This vessel left Blackwall on October 20th of that year, and rather more than a month later put in at Priok, Batavia, for coaling. No cargo was taken on board, only fresh vegetables and fruit were obtained for the saloon table. Distilled water from condensers was used throughout the voyage, and no water was shipped at Priok. A case of cholera (with somewhat doubtful symptoms) occurred on board four days after leaving Priok; the patient recovered. Seven days afterwards an unmistakable case presented itself, with a fatal result in twelve hours. From December 10th to 23rd there were other cases, and in all seventeen deaths. None of the officers, crew, or saloon passengers were attacked. The saloon passengers had landed at Priok, and passed the night there. It was well known that cholera was then epidemic in Batavia. The belief was entertained by the ship's officers that the infection existed in some sand brought on board at Priok for the purpose of cleansing the decks. This sand was very black, and imparted a peculiarly offensive smell to water. It was used only for two days, around the berths of the single and married men, and then thrown away.

In this case there was no ground for supposing that the drinking water had become polluted. The fact that the disease occurred only among the steerage passengers was somewhat curious. Some of these, however, had gone on shore at Priok, and all had eaten more or less fruit, which they bought for themselves —probably in great abundance, as it was very cheap. It is difficult to estimate the degree of probability attaching to the view that the infective material was contained in the sand and taken into the system through the lungs. Such a mode of communication cannot be regarded as *impossible*, especially if credit is to be given to the following account of a case in which other channels of infection seemed to be wanting.

On March 28th, 1866, the steamship *England* left Liverpool with about one thousand two hundred passengers for Halifax. Cholera broke out five days afterwards, and carried off some three hundred persons. As the ship bore up for Halifax, she was hailed by a pilot who was cruising in a boat with two other men; he agreed to bring the ship into the quarantine harbour at Halifax, and, having been told that there was a fatal disease on board, laid his boat alongside, sent up his papers to the captain in a basket that had been lowered from the ship, and was then taken in tow. Having brought the ship up to the quarantine harbour, *without having boarded her*, he rowed ashore with his two comrades. On the night of April 10th, or two days after he had thus come remotely into contact with the *England*, he was taken ill with cholera, and three days afterwards cholera broke out in his family. Almost at the same time one of his two companions sickened, and gave the disease to his three children. According to statements in the Army Medical Reports for that year, the whole Western hemisphere was at that time, and had been for years, quite free from cholera.

The discovery of the essential and specific cause of cholera would go far to determine many questions regarding the spread and propagation of the disease. An account of the controversies which have taken place on this subject would fill a large volume. In the minds of the speculative, the disease has been vaguely associated with astral influences, the approach of comets, various meteorological phenomena, the presence of ozone in the air, peculiar electrical states of the atmosphere, mists of various colours, etc. No facts, however, exist to prove anything more than a merely accidental connection between any of these circumstances and the appearance of cholera, and nothing certainly to authorise the suspicion that they stand towards each other in the relation of cause and effect.

The theory that cholera is due to invisible animalcules was advanced many decades ago, and was supported by many facts connected with the outbreak and spread of the disease. Nearly fifty years ago Pacini alleged that he had discovered such organisms; but his observations turned out to be valueless. In 1884 Dr. Koch stated that the causal agent of Asiatic cholera was a peculiar species of bacterium, which can always be demonstrated in the intestinal contents and in the dejecta of persons suffering from the disease. It is not found in the intestinal contents of healthy persons, nor in those suffering from other diseases; it is exclusively confined to the cholera intestine, and its numbers are directly proportionate to the severity of the attack.

Koch's theory, based on his discovery of the micro-organisms, is now almost universally accepted. Our knowledge of the life-history of the bacilli found in cholera patients is, however, far from being complete. We know that these micro-organisms take the form of minute curved rods, the largest among them measuring only $\frac{1}{12000}$th of an inch in length, whilst the smallest are less than half this size. Only those persons who are conversant with the use of the microscope can form a proper idea of such minuteness. Sometimes a dozen or more organisms are united together so as to form a long screw-shaped thread.

These bacilli are vegetable parasites, which increase and multiply within the body to an enormous extent, and with marvellous rapidity. With regard to the nature and mode of growth, and multiplication of bacteria in general, we know that these organisms are exceedingly minute plants, some of which live as parasites within the human body. They multiply by fission or simple division, and in some species by the formation of spores or seeds. These latter are highly important, inasmuch as they possess greater powers of resistance and stronger vitality than the parent organism, so that the continuance of the species is effected by them, from one season to another, under conditions which would destroy the fully formed parasite. Bacteria, as a rule, are killed by a temperature of about 212° Fahr. The spores, however, of some species require a temperature of 250° to 270° Fahr. to destroy them completely; hence ordinary boiling is far from being sufficient.

Many species of bacteria—*e.g.*, those which cause fermentation—are altogether innocuous, so far as man is concerned, but others are the direct causes of disease. It has been suggested that those belonging to the second class are the result of transformation of innocent forms, that they have been evolved by a process of natural selection. According to this view, the infective bacteria have not always possessed their noxious qualities, but have acquired them somehow in the course of ages. It is certain that such changes would require long periods for their production; but in view of the modifications of virulence which can be artificially caused in the micro-organisms of several diseases, the theory of transformation must be regarded as not altogether improbable.

We have no definite knowledge as to the manner in which the bacteria set up the phenomena of disease. In some cases they have an obvious local action; in others they cause general symptoms, such as fever and wasting; in a third class both forms of action are manifested. The mischief wrought, of whatever kind it may be, is not the result of mere contact. It would appear that the living organisms secrete or produce a poison which is conveyed through the fluids of the tissues, and is the cause of the local and general changes. This explanation is supported by the rapid poisoning sometimes witnessed after animals are inoculated with anthrax. Death may occur within twenty-four hours, though the organisms are, by that time, very sparingly diffused. The fatal result is due to poison, doubtless produced by the organisms, but not as yet isolated.

But to return to the bacilli of cholera. One important part of their life-history is wanting, for no spore-formation has been clearly observed, and their mode of multiplication is as yet doubtful. The spores of some kinds of bacilli, when dried, retain their vitality for months or years; those which may be produced by the micro-organism of cholera do not possess this property. It is stated that if fluids containing cholera bacilli, or linen impregnated with them, once become dry, no further development can be brought about under the most favourable circumstances. If this assertion be correct, we must adopt the conclusion that no living cholera bacilli can be contained in any material which is in a dry or dust-like state; and as it is only from completely dry surfaces that particles of dust can be detached and carried to other localities by currents of air, it follows that the transport of living cholera bacilli by the air, and the production of infection in this way, are impossible (Flügge). It is, however, admitted that cholera bacilli may be transported through the air for short distances when infective fluids are agitated and bubbles are detached, as, for instance, when waves strike against a quay or on the wheels of a water-mill, or when the soiled linen of cholera patients is being washed; in these cases small bubbles of fluid containing bacilli may be brought by currents of air into contact with predisposed individuals.

The statements above quoted are founded upon the results of many experiments frequently repeated, and conducted with the greatest care. The bacilli are cultivated in suitable media, and their behaviour is watched under various conditions. It may be that all the natural circumstances favourable to the growth and development of cholera bacilli have not as yet been ascertained and imitated. The conditions which promote their increase in water have been very closely studied. The fluid must contain organic material in solution, and not exhibit any acid reaction. Meat infusion and milk are very suitable media. It was alleged that in the Hamburg epidemic the substances used to disinfect the river really promoted the development of the cholera bacilli, inasmuch as they killed large numbers of fish, which, undergoing decomposition, supplied an abundance of organic material to the water.

A few words as to the measures to be taken to arrest the spread of cholera. We must act upon the theory that the disease is communicable, and that it is disseminated chiefly or exclusively by the dejections of cholera patients. Recent experience distinctly shows that drinking water is the vehicle by which the poison most often gains access to the body. It may remain an open question whether the poison ever rises into the air with the products of evaporation, or whether it ever passes into a dry state and takes the form of impalpable dust. To make security as complete as possible, it is well to regard these latter modes of communication as at least not improbable.

The precautions to be taken may be divided into two classes—special and general.

1. When cholera has once broken out in a given locality, it is only natural that the inhabitants of adjacent places should take steps to prevent invasion. Human beings are the carriers of the germs of the disease, and if the affected spot or district could be completely cut off from all communication with its neighbours, the progress of the disease would doubtless be arrested. Absolutely rigid quarantine is, however, usually impossible, and events have

shown that it is not essentially necessary. The strictest watch should, however, be exercised over every possible channel of communication, and all persons coming from an infected country should be carefully examined. Even if they be found healthy, a short detention, perhaps for three or four days, may often be desirable. There is, however, much doubt as to the length of the incubation period of cholera, that is, the time which elapses between infection and the appearance of the earliest symptoms. Mr. Macnamara's cases show that twenty-four hours may be sufficient; but Dr. Parkes states that this stage can certainly last for ten or twelve days, and that there are some good cases on record where it lasted for more than twenty. Quarantine, therefore, unless enforced for at least three weeks, might be quite useless.

When cases of cholera already exist, every endeavour should be made to destroy, by means of disinfectants or by burning, the poisonous properties of the dejecta from patients. Corrosive sublimate is the best destructive, and a solution containing one part in 1,000 of water should be added freely to the discharges. A solution of carbolic acid (1 to 20 water) is now recommended as more efficacious. Another good plan is to mix the discharges with dry sawdust and sulphur, and to burn with a sufficiency of straw and wood. The bedding, body linen, and other articles tainted with the discharges should be either burnt or soaked for some hours in the sublimate, or carbolic acid solution, and afterwards exposed to the action of super-heated steam. The attendants on the sick should observe the most scrupulous cleanliness, and should be careful to wash their hands with hot water, soap, sand, and disinfectants immediately after performing the necessary offices for the sick. If it be impossible to burn the discharges, they should, after disinfection, be buried deeply in the soil, as far as possible from wells and other sources of water supply.

The purity of the water used for drinking is a matter of supreme importance. In country places, where cesspools and wells are sometimes not many yards apart, the danger of polluted water is very great. Moreover, shallow wells (*i.e.*, less than fifty feet deep) not passing through impermeable strata, as stiff clay or hard rock, are especially dangerous. The drainage of the neighbouring land tends towards them, and heavy rains will often wash many substances into them. It has been proved that cholera bacilli soon perish in *pure* water; but if organic matters be present, rapid multiplication is the rule. In addition to passing through a filter, all suspected water should be previously boiled. There is good reason for believing that domestic filters too often fail to answer any good purpose; indeed, in some cases, their action is directly mischievous. This result is due to the impure state into which the filtering material is allowed to get. It seems to be forgotten that filters act by keeping back injurious particles, which in the course of time accumulate in the interstices and on the surface of the filtering material. Unless the latter is from time to time cleansed or renewed, fairly good water may actually take up impurities from the filter. If charcoal be used as a filtering agent, it should be boiled from time to time, say once a month, and then dried by exposure to the sun, or in an oven. A charcoal ball should be well scraped, and allowed to remain for some time in hot water. The spongy iron filters are perhaps the best for general use; the material is cheap, and can be easily renewed. The Chamberland-Pasteur filters, as described in the essay on the London Water Supply, are said to be remarkably efficacious in preventing the passage of micro-organisms.

It is almost needless to add that water should never be allowed to remain in cisterns, unless the latter are easily accessible and are kept perfectly clean. No drinking water should be drawn from a cistern which is in direct communication with a pipe employed for flushing a closet.

In view of the fact that the cholera poison is conveyed by water, the inhabitants of London may be congratulated on the withdrawal of the proposal to provide a hospital for cholera patients on the Thames at Blackfriars. Facility of access is the only recommendation attaching to such a plan; but this is altogether outweighed by the terrible risk necessarily involved.

2. The general rules for the prevention of cholera are those of ordinary hygiene. The cholera poison multiplies only under insanitary

conditions; it fails to obtain a footing wherever the laws of health are observed. Filth in any form, and especially earth sodden with animal dejections and refuse, favour the development of such diseases as cholera and typhoid, and render individuals more liable to become affected. Hence all drains, closets, etc., should be kept in perfect order; fresh air should be admitted as freely as possible into every room; dampness of the surrounding soil should be remedied, and the most scrupulous cleanliness should be observed. Moderation and care in such matters as eating, drinking, and exercise decidedly tend to lessen the danger of contagion. Excessive indulgence in alcoholic liquors could only render the system more liable to attack. It is sometimes, though erroneously, supposed that the addition of ardent spirits to water destroys or neutralises impurities. Unripe fruit and indigestible food, as tending to cause irritation of the abdominal organs, should be scrupulously avoided. Chills are likely to be mischievous; an extra layer of thin flannel or silk round the waist may be worn with advantage. Medical advice should be sought on the first appearance of diarrhœa.

A few words must be added on the method of preventing attacks of cholera by inoculating with an attenuated virus persons likely to be exposed to contagion. The method, which has been brought to a high degree of perfection by M. Haffkine, is based on knowledge gained from laboratory experience. The cholera virus, capable of causing the severest form of the disease, is gradually transformed into one which, though almost or quite harmless, protects inoculated persons in a greater or less degree. This anti-cholera vaccination, so-called, has now been applied to thousands of persons in India, and the accumulated evidence is decidedly in its favour. There is, of course, some difference of opinion as to its utility; but if the experiments be continued during another year or two, and the results still prove highly favourable, it is difficult to imagine that any ground will remain for scepticism.

More than twenty-five years have elapsed since any epidemic of cholera has raged in this country. During that interval the disease has reached our ports, but has failed to establish a footing. We may fairly attribute this immunity to the improved sanitary conditions which now obtain in all our large towns. We cannot be too thankful for this result, and we ought not to neglect its obvious lessons. In country places much remains to be done in order to bring the sanitary conditions to a level with our knowledge. We cannot plead ignorance; apathy and indifference are the foes most to be dreaded.

X.

INFECTION AND DISINFECTION.

THE enormous variety of subjects contained in medical literature necessitates the use of a corresponding number of terms, the majority of which have a certain and well-known meaning, but it would be difficult to find two words more wanting in the element of precision and more loosely used than those placed at the head of this article. The general public, indeed, solve all difficulties by connecting with the word "infection" the idea of something "catching"—*i.e.*, something that can be propagated from one person to another, and disinfection is correspondingly regarded as the means whereby such propagation can be hindered. It must be admitted that this simple view is quite correct so far as it goes. It of course disregards all questions as to the nature of infection, and the reason why some diseases spread from person to person and others do not, and it included the belief that disinfection is generally attainable, and by comparatively simple means. In cases especially where the use of some well-advertised material is found to neutralise or mask an unpleasant odour, the completeness of the disinfection is looked upon as absolutely certain.

In medical writings the confusion has been still further increased by the use of the words "contagion" and "contagious" in describing those diseases which were considered to spread from one person to another by contact. "Infection" and "infectious" were limited to the cases in which the poison of the disease was supposed to be conveyed by the atmosphere from the sick person to those at a greater or less distance from him. Accordingly, we used to hear of a disease being contagious but not infectious, and *vice versâ*. The distinction is, however, a purely artificial one, and is not sustained by facts; for many of the contagious diseases can be propagated indirectly, that is, without actual contact between the person who yields the poison and the person who receives it. Take, for example, diphtheria; it assuredly spreads by contact, and is therefore contagious, and no less positively is the poison capable of being disseminated through the atmosphere and infecting those who inhale it. So, too, with small-pox. If its virus be introduced under the skin of a person unprotected by vaccination or a previous attack, he will almost certainly suffer from the disease, and the same result would follow were such a person to be in close attendance upon a small-pox patient. In the latter case, the poison floating about in the atmosphere would get into the system through the lungs, and this is practically just as much an example of *contact* as if the poison were artificially introduced through the skin. It is therefore better to consider the terms "infection" and "contagion" as practically synonymous, and they will be so used in the remarks that follow.

To show what is implied by an infectious disease, let me take a typical example and contrast it with another disorder well known to be non-infectious. A young adult, previously in good health, is suddenly attacked by such symptoms as chilliness, soreness of throat, and evidences of derangement of the stomach.

There is nothing characteristic about these symptoms; but let us suppose that on the following day there is high fever, dryness of skin, headache, giddiness, etc., and that in a few hours a scarlet rash appears, first on the chest, and then spreads over the body. All the symptoms become worse, and for ten or twelve days the patient is very ill. After this period, in favourable cases, a change takes place for the better, the rash dies away, and all the other symptoms gradually subside. In from three to six weeks, supposing that there are no complications, the patient regards himself as well. Such, in a few words, is the course of a mild case of scarlet fever, which may be considered as a typically infectious disease. Now suppose that our patient is treated in a house where there are several other young people who have never suffered from the disease. We know from experience that unless the most minute precautions are taken, the majority of these persons will exhibit similar symptoms. It is also well known that if any of these patients, supposed to have partially recovered from the disease, change their place of abode and go among other friends, the latter will run great risk of being attacked, and that the disease may thus spread *ad infinitum*. This capacity of propagation, the possession of which is as certain as anything can possibly be, suggests the inquiry as to the manner in which the original patient of our series became infected. He in his turn must have taken the disease from some one else, but it is quite possible that he has never been within a mile of a scarlet fever patient. In many such instances it is impossible to get any clue to the original case; but it sometimes happens that evidence is forthcoming to the effect that days or weeks, or even months before, a person convalescent from the disease had occupied a room of which our patient was afterwards a tenant, or that some article of clothing which once belonged to patient number one had been handled or worn by the person whose case we are considering. It is evident that there must often be great difficulties in prosecuting such an inquiry.

Let us now take an example of a non-infectious disease, and notice how it contrasts with the one we have just described. A young adult, previously in good health, becomes sensible of a feeling of heat alternating with chilliness and perhaps shivering, and slight pains in the limbs. In a day or two there is more or less fever and thirst, and some of the larger joints are swollen and very painful, while the skin covering them is much reddened. The pain and fever are the principal symptoms; but there are often others, a description of which is unnecessary for our present purpose. The complaint lasts an indefinite time, but even in the absence of treatment usually subsides within six weeks. Such, in a very few words, is the course of rheumatic fever or acute rheumatism.

These two diseases—scarlet fever and rheumatic fever—have much in common, but there are sharp points of difference between them. In both fever is a prominent symptom, and in addition to the display of local symptoms the whole system is evidently affected. The differences, however, are still more important. Scarlet fever is eminently infectious. The air which surrounds the patient becomes contaminated and highly charged with the poison, and persons breathing it run great risk of becoming affected. In a case of rheumatic fever, although the secretion from the skin is generally very copious and peculiar in character, so that the sense of smell is strongly appealed to, there is no such risk; the disease cannot be conveyed from the patient to those around him, however close the attendance and however defective the ventilation of the room. Infection from a previous case is therefore never thought of in connection with rheumatic fever, though the actual nature of the poison which causes the disease is as yet unknown. The attack is often excited by exposure to cold and wet, circumstances which play no part in the causation of scarlet fever. There is at least one more important difference between the two diseases: scarlet fever very rarely indeed occurs a second time in the same patient, and the symptoms never become chronic; rheumatic fever, on the other hand, is very prone to recur, and in not a few cases the original attack merges into a chronic state of suffering, which may continue for months or even years.

I have taken scarlet fever as a representative of the class of infectious diseases the cause of which is the contamination of the system by some specific poison, and I have sketched in a few words the main symptoms which result. For our present purposes the important points are the contagious or infectious character of the disease, and the proofs that the contagious material multiplies within the system which it has invaded, and from which it sallies forth in quest of other victims. There are, unfortunately, not a few diseases belonging to the same category as scarlet fever, the principal being small-pox, measles, typhus, influenza, whooping-cough, diphtheria, typhoid, and cholera. With regard to all these it may be stated that they are quite separate and distinct as regards causation. A case of scarlet fever never gives rise to small-pox in those exposed to infection, neither does any one of the above diseases ever pass into another. There are other subordinate distinctions: the poison of scarlet fever, contained presumably in detached particles of skin, clings for months to articles of clothing, especially woollen ones; that of small-pox may be collected from the eruption and preserved for years between pieces of glass; that of typhus is easily rendered innocuous by free ventilation. All these peculiarities—and many more might be cited—point to important differences in the nature of the infectious materials.

What this infectious material really is has often been keenly debated since medicine became a science, and at the present time is the question which most closely occupies the minds of medical investigators. Merely to enumerate the inquiries and to describe the experiments and the theories based thereon would fill many volumes; but it is not to be wondered at that this subject should have excited so much attention when we reflect upon the prevalence and fatality of the diseases in question, and upon the comparatively slight influence which treatment exercises upon their course. On the other hand, experience clearly shows that their prevention is not only possible, but in some cases easily accomplished. The knowledge of the causes of these diseases would indicate the proper preventive measures, or at any rate the direction which such measures should take, and hence a discovery of the cause in any given case at once yields practical results.

When we know what causes infection we can apply disinfection with every prospect of success. Without such knowledge, success if attained must be accidental rather than otherwise. The nature of the contagious agencies and the medium through which they spread are the most important points in connection with the subject of infection.

There is strong evidence in support of the view that these contagia are actual living things. Formerly the opinion was universally held that infectious diseases were caused by foul air ; and the effluvia connected with putrid decomposition were regarded as a sufficient cause for the development of fever, small-pox, etc. It cannot be denied that gaseous matters, notably sulphuretted hydrogen, may act as poisons and cause many serious symptoms, but it has never been shown that infectious diseases originate in this manner. It is contrary to all that chemistry teaches us that sulphuretted hydrogen or ammoniacal vapours inhaled by the lungs should increase within the body and cause it to become a centre of infection ; and we know likewise that ordinary poisons—*e.g.*, arsenic or morphia—

fatal as their effects may be to one individual, have no power of increase and propagation after being once taken. It is therefore evident that the poisons of infectious diseases must be something of an entirely different nature. We know that they multiply in the system to an almost infinite extent, and that every one of the myriads of atoms thus developed is as potent for evil as the atom from which it originated. The possession of this and other properties clearly indicates that the contagious agencies are independent living organisms capable of growth and reproduction. It has long been known that certain diseases of the skin—*e.g.*, ringworm—are caused by the presence of parasites which very rapidly increase, and can be easily recognised under the microscrope.

In the case of some three or four of the infectious diseases it would seem that the poison has really been discovered. On examining vaccine matter, the contents of the pocks in small-pox, and discharges in glanders, the microscope shows a vast number of infinitely minute particles, which appear as glistening points. Some of these are even less than the fifty-thousandth of an inch in diameter, and it therefore follows that very high powers are necessary for their detection. Such particles, obtained from vaccine lymph, have been washed in water; the water when inoculated did not produce any effect, but the washed particles were found to have retained their potency. It seems fair to infer that the contagious agents of the other infective diseases would resemble in their physical characters that of vaccine, and the nature of such particles is the important problem that offers itself for solution. They are supposed by some, and notably by Dr. Beale, to be of animal origin, and to consist of elementary living matter, termed *bioplasm*. Such particles may be easily transferred from an infected to an uninfected organism, in which they will manifest their own specific powers, and grow and multiply almost indefinitely, exciting in their new home a series of changes resembling those which characterised their presence in the one from which they were derived. This account is certainly correct as regards the virus of vaccine, but it does not precisely define the nature of the particles or tell us anything of their origin. Dr. Beale, however, states that particles of contagious bioplasm are not generated in the organism of the infected animal, but are introduced from without, and were originally derived by direct descent from the bioplasm of the body of man or animal. He regards them, in fact, as particles of degraded bioplasm. This theory is not in favour at the present time. One objection to its validity is constituted by the fact that particles of living animal matter die very rapidly after they have escaped from the body, whereas many contagious germs preserve their vitality and capacity for evil for a very long time.

Another theory which was promulgated some twenty years ago was to the effect that the contagious particles are of the nature of those low vegetable organisms which are termed *fungi*. This view gains support from the manner in which these bodies increase in number when planted in a suitable soil, and the power which they possess of decomposing many organic substances. The fact, already referred to, that several diseases of the skin and hair in men and animals are undoubtedly due to fungi, also tends to recommend this theory. Recent experiments, however, have shown that these organisms, capable as some of them are of growth and development on the *surface* of the body, do not possess the power of growth and reproduction *within* the body, and it is therefore unlikely that they should be the causes of disease in which the system is charged with poisonous materials.

A third theory is one which is extremely popular at the present day, advocated as it is by investigators of the highest repute. It is almost needless to say that I refer to the view which credits certain minute organisms, termed *bacteria*, with the power of causing the infectious diseases—that is, with being in themselves the poisonous agents. So firm is the hold that this view has obtained that "disease-germs" and "bacteria" are used as though they were synonymous terms. It is, moreover, probable that more experiments have been made with reference to bacteria than on any other subject whatever.

The term "bacterium" signifies a rod, and many of these organisms are minute rod-shaped bodies. They or their germs are very widely diffused throughout nature; they swarm in the air and in water, especially if containing organic matter, and are likewise found in great numbers within the bodies of men and animals. Any one who possesses a microscope with a magnifying power of five hundred diameters can readily examine a very common form of bacterium. It is only necessary to take a glass of ordinary water from a spring or river, and to leave it in a warm room exposed for some days to the air. A thin coating, looking like a deposit of fine dust, is formed on the surface of the water; this dust consists of myriads of bacteria, which are readily seen when a drop of the water is examined. The bacteria are found to be in several stages of transformation: some are in long jointed rods, others represent one or more detached portions of these rods, and others appear as extremely minute rounded particles. Some of the rods are capable of movement, and are seen to wriggle through the fluid like small eels or snakes. The minute rounded particles are the spores, which eventually become rod-shaped bodies. These and other organisms are found in great abundance in an infusion of hay, set aside for some days till it has become turbid. They are present in vast numbers wherever there is putrefaction.

The peculiar interest connected with these simple experiments is due to the fact that minute organisms closely resembling those just described are found in the bodies of patients suffering from acute infectious diseases, and the question naturally arises as to the relation which exists between the organisms and the symptoms. Are the former the cause of the latter, or is their presence a mere coincidence? Another suggestion is that their presence is the result of the disease. If the symptoms are really caused by the presence and action of the bacteria, it would follow that differences must exist between the organisms found in different diseases. Great and manifold difficulties attend such investigations; it is sufficient here to notice the extreme minuteness of the organisms, necessitating the use of the highest powers of the microscope for their detection. Moreover, as already stated, bacteria are found in large numbers in the bodies of persons apparently healthy, and some of these organisms very closely resemble, if indeed they are not identical with, those that have been found in connection with severe infectious diseases. It is hardly conceivable that minute organisms which abound, for example, in the mouth and give rise to no changes, should be capable in other parts of causing the most serious symptoms.

In order to prove that a micro-organism is the real cause of a disease, at least three conditions must be fulfilled. In the first place, the same species of micro-organism must be invariably found in the blood, lymph, or diseased tissue of man or animal suffering from or dead of the disease. Secondly, the organism must be cultivated apart from the body in which it has been found, so as to make sure that it has been separated from all other morbid materials to the presence of which the disease might possibly be due. Thirdly, when the organisms thus cultivated have been introduced into the body of an animal capable of being attacked by the disease, similar symptoms ought to be set up, and the same micro-organisms should be found in the newly affected animal. If, in testing any given disease, these conditions are fulfilled, it is scarcely possible to doubt that the micro-organisms are the cause; they certainly cannot be the result. It is fair, also, to argue from diseases in which the conditions are fulfilled, that others in which, owing to circumstances, the tests cannot be properly carried out are due to similar causes.

Very strong evidence is forthcoming in support of the theory that micro-organisms are the cause of infectious diseases. Horned cattle and sheep are subject to a disease termed anthrax, or splenic fever; and so far back as 1849, minute rod-shaped bodies were found in the blood of animals which had died from this disease, which is also communicable to man. The significance of these rods was suspected only after Pasteur's researches into the part played by minute organisms in fermentation. Guided by these discoveries, Davaine inoculated healthy animals with blood from those diseased, with the result of producing similar symptoms, while myriads of organisms were found in the bodies of those animals which had been inoculated with a very minute quantity of blood. The symptoms are very characteristic, and the disease at one time caused an enormous mortality among cattle in France. By the opponents of the bacterium hypothesis it might of course be urged that in the inoculation experiments other morbid materials were simultaneously conveyed and that the transmission of the disease was due to their presence.

To meet this objection, and to fulfil the second condition laid down in the last paragraph, experiments for cultivating the organisms were set on foot in the following manner. A drop of blood taken from an animal that had died from anthrax was put into a glass flask containing an infusion of yeast, which had been carefully treated and proved to be free from organisms. In twenty-four hours the liquid, previously clear, was seen to be full of very light flakes, which, when examined under the microscope, were found to be masses of organisms resembling those contained in the blood. A drop taken from this first flask was added to a second, and produced the same effect, and a drop from this was added to a third, and so on till a tenth flask was thus charged with organisms. In this way the organisms were enormously multiplied and completely freed from the admixture of any other substance. Yet when a drop was taken from the twentieth or even the fiftieth flask of such a series, and inserted under the skin of a sheep, it caused anthrax or splenic fever, attended by the same symptoms as those produced by the drop of blood taken from the first animal. It is impossible to conceive of any clearer proof that the organisms are the sole cause of the disease. So crucial a test, however, cannot be applied in every case; for many of the infectious diseases which are the scourge of mankind do not affect the lower animals, and it is therefore impossible to make trial of the organisms found in connection therewith. Besides anthrax, there are other infective diseases in animals which have been proved to be due to bacteria, and these facts strongly support the belief that the infectious diseases of mankind are due to the invasion of similar organisms. It is, however, impossible as yet to dogmatise upon this subject. There have already been too many assertions and inferences drawn therefrom which have turned out to be unwarranted. It is comparatively easy for skilled observers to detect the presence of micro-organisms, and whenever uniformity of appearance is demonstrable in connection with a given disease, a decided addition has been made to our knowledge. For reasons above given, the next point—viz., the determining whether the organisms are the cause of the disease, is surrounded with great difficulties. The discoveries, however, with regard to splenic fever strongly support the view that bacteria are the efficient agents of contagious diseases.

Space will not permit me to do more than allude to the various theories that have been advanced with regard to the manner in which these tiny organisms produce disease. It was at first thought that they acted like parasites, and exhausted the system during their development. It is now, however, more commonly believed that the organisms elaborate a special ferment or poison, which, when produced in sufficient amount, gives rise to the symptoms of the disease.

One of the most valuable results of the study of these organisms is the discovery that, by cultivation, the virulence of some, at least, can be so mitigated that when inoculated they produce only slight and non-fatal symptoms, the development of which in a given animal is nevertheless protective against future attacks of the original disease. By cultivating the organisms of splenic fever at a temperature of 108° it is found that filaments are produced, but not spores, and that by repeated cultivation this growth becomes altered as regards its properties of causing disease. When inoculated, it sets up a mild form of splenic fever, not dangerous to life, but perfectly protective against subsequent inoculation with the otherwise poisonous organisms. This discovery is worthy of being classed with that of vaccination as a protection against small-pox.

The immunity acquired by protective inoculation is a very interesting and important subject. As a result of Pasteur's successful experiments upon fowl-cholera and splenic fever, the idea naturally arose that all infectious diseases might be prevented by antecedent inoculation with attenuated virus. This expectation, however, is not likely to be altogether fulfilled; for we know that in the case of some infectious diseases—small-pox, for example—even a first attack does not always protect the patient against a second. But such cases are quite exceptional, and the conclusion to be drawn from the results of Pasteur's method, modified and adapted to various diseases by other investigators, are such as to justify the utmost confidence in "protective inoculation." As a further development of experimental researches, it has been found that the watery portion (the serum) of the blood of animals rendered immune is, as regards some diseases, capable of conferring immunity upon other animals. The infection of the poisonous products of bacteria leads to the development in the blood of substances to which the term "antitoxin" has been applied. These substances are found to be "protective"; they neutralise or destroy the injected poison, and the fluid thus rendered "antitoxic" can be used to protect other animals. As related in the chapter on diphtheria, there is every reason to hope that an "antitoxin" has been discovered the use of which will greatly reduce the mortality caused by that widespread disease.

With regard to the channels through which the contagious organisms are spread, a few words will suffice to state what is known on this point, which is intimately connected with the subject of disinfection. Air and water are the chief media for the propagation of infectious disease. In the case of scarlet fever, which has been taken as the type, the scales detached from the skin, and similar tissues from the throat, contain the germs of the disease, and these find their way into the atmosphere and are received into the lungs. They attach themselves also to articles of clothing and furniture, and are thus often carried to long distances. The tenacity with which such contagia adhere to woollen articles is very remarkable. Sir Thomas Watson relates the following instance:—A house in which several persons had been attacked by scarlet fever was left empty for a year. When the family returned, a drawer in one of the bedrooms resisted for some time attempts to pull it open. A strip of flannel had got between the drawer and its frame, and had made the drawer stick. This piece of flannel the housemaid put playfully round her neck. An old nurse who was present, recognising it as having been used as an application to the throat of one of the subjects of scarlet fever, snatched it away and burnt it. The girl, however, soon sickened with the disease. In the cases of cholera and typhoid fever, the discharges from the patient find their way into water, which thus becomes the channel by which the diseases are propagated. Food, too, may become similarly contaminated. Milk, for instance, has been often known to convey the poisons of typhoid fever, of scarlet fever, and of diphtheria. In the case of the first, the contamination has been probably due to adulterating the milk with foul water containing the disease-germs, but it may have arisen in some cases from the typhoid emanations having been absorbed by the milk. The poisons of scarlet fever and diphtheria were probably transmitted to the milk from the skins and throats of persons employed in the dairy, and recently convalescent or scarcely recovered from attacks of these diseases. The germs of certain other infectious diseases find their way into the system through abraded surfaces of the body.

The fatal character of many infectious

diseases, and the ease and rapidity with which they spread and attack large masses of the population, are sufficient to account for the endeavours that have been made since very early times to arrest their progress. As in many other matters, practice has preceded science, and centuries before the vaguest ideas were entertained as to the nature of the diseases which seemed destined to be the scourges of mankind, efforts were made to stamp them out. As might be expected, many of these efforts were of the rudest description, but the earliest of them aimed at the object which the most modern science also seeks to achieve—viz., the destruction of the contagious material. The term "disinfection" first occurred in literature towards the end of the last century. A French writer, Morveau, in 1801, published a work on "The Disinfection of the Air," but the word was used somewhat earlier by a few English writers.

The most ancient method consisted in destroying by fire everything that had been in contact with the source of infection, the idea, no doubt, being that as fire consumes what is visible, it likewise destroys what is invisible. It is possible that the practice of burning the dead was in a measure based upon the conviction that a source of danger to the living was thus got rid of. The thirteenth chapter of Leviticus contains the most minute directions for disinfecting cases of leprosy; destruction of suspected articles by means of fire, the copious use of water, and isolation of the leper, are the means prescribed. Inspection by the priest was to decide as to the efficacy of these measures. Among the Egyptians and certain Asiatic peoples, the fumigations used by the priests in exorcising disease were probably neither more nor less efficacious than similar processes in vogue at the present day in some European countries.

In the growth of ideas with regard to the causes of infectious diseases, the theory gradually took shape that the infecting matters were formed as a result of the processes of decomposition; and as these processes are generally attended with the development of more or less unpleasant odours, it seemed only natural to assume that the causes of the latter were also the causes of disease. In addition to regarding foul emanations as generally mischievous, the idea was entertained that there was something quite specific about them, and accordingly we find that attempts to mask or neutralise them were regarded as the best methods of checking the spread of infectious diseases. Deodorisation came to be considered as equivalent to disinfection. The idea was the more welcome inasmuch as it could be carried into effect without destroying property and without much difficulty. The attempt was certainly in the right direction, for the destruction of noxious agencies was the object in view. Unfortunately the means employed absolutely failed to effect their purpose, and belief in their efficacy caused very mischievous results—viz., a sense of false security and neglect of ventilation and cleanliness as regards sick persons and surrounding objects. In fact, the confident adoption of deodorants as a means of checking the spread of infectious diseases was a decidedly retrograde step as compared with the use of fire for destruction and of water as a purifying agent.

Chlorine gas was the deodorant which came into very general use at the beginning of the present century. It was freely employed in hospitals, both civil and military, in prisons, workhouses, etc., and was supposed to be efficacious against fevers, cholera, and small-pox. Whenever its characteristic odour could be perceived, danger of infection was no longer feared. Persons carried about with them small flasks containing chemicals which generated this gas, and inhaled a little when they considered themselves exposed to risk. It soon, however, became evident that these precautions were useless; but even so recently as 1866, during the war between Austria and Prussia, it was thought sufficient to distribute saucers containing chloride of lime throughout the military hospitals, while only feeble efforts were made to ensure cleanliness and other important sanitary requirements. In order to act as a real disinfectant, chlorine must be employed in a very different manner. The terrible mortality after surgical operations and severe injuries—a feature of which was that a large majority of patients died with symptoms of blood-poisoning—showed the futility of such attempts at disinfection.

In spite, however, of many similar failures,

deodorisation has been almost universally regarded as the main object to be accomplished, and other chemical agents have been used in order to combat the gaseous products of decomposition. This object could certainly be attained if the sense of smell were to be the sole judge of success; and the practice of deodorisation led also to the discovery and use of many substances which have the power to prevent or retard putrefaction, and were therefore termed antiseptics, and regarded as equivalent to disinfectants. The conclusion, however, was soon forced upon the minds of experimenters that the infective agencies of fevers, small-pox, etc., were neither offensive gases nor the products of putrefaction, but something of an entirely different character. When an infectious disease became associated with the idea of a transportable material which increases and multiplies in its new ground, the discovery was not far off that organisms capable of reproduction are the real causes of the disease.

Definite ideas now prevail as to what is meant by disinfection, and as to the methods by which this object can be attained and the tests whereby their efficacy may be proved. Any substance may be regarded as a true disinfectant which, when added to a quantity of fluid swarming with bacteria, abolishes the reproductive power of these organisms. If the bacteria are capable of producing disease, or the poison of disease, a successful experiment has been made in the way of disinfection. This fact explains the paucity of the real experiences we possess of disinfection proper. Heat, exposure to air and sunlight, removal by mechanical processes, and the use of chemical agencies, are the means at our disposal; it will be sufficient to point out a few of the methods in which they may be employed.

A very high temperature, say of 240° and upwards, will, of course, destroy all such forms of organised matter as we are now considering, and if we could always isolate the germs of disease, and expose them to great heat, the task of disinfection would be thoroughly accomplished. Such isolation is of course impossible; but we make use of heat for the destruction of germs which have found a resting-place in clothes, bedding, and textile articles of furniture. The application of heat requires apparatus which cannot be extemporised, and which are indeed beyond the capacity of private resources. The infected articles have to be placed in ovens or hot-air chambers, the temperature of which can be raised many degrees above the boiling-point of water. A high temperature, however, has less effect upon the spores than upon the mature organisms, but successive heatings are found to effect the desired result. During their development, which is much promoted by the influence of heat, the spores rapidly pass through several stages, in which they become softened and far more capable of final destruction. Exposure to a current of steam at a temperature of 212° is a more potent, rapid, and satisfactory method than the use of dry heat, and it has the further advantage of causing less injury to the articles to be disinfected. This question of injury to infected articles is of much importance in dealing with poor patients; but under different circumstances, or when the articles are of small value, complete destruction by fire is the best means of disposing of them. In the majority of cases, and especially when the articles consist of blankets and other woollen goods, destruction has to be avoided, and the problem to be solved is how to disinfect thoroughly and at the same time do as little damage as possible to the textures. Those materials which are derived from the animal kingdom are the most expensive and the most difficult to deal with, and are at the same time the favourite resting-places of the germs of disease, which, when contained in woollen materials, are protected from currents of air and thus preserved. As Dr. Russell, the Medical Officer of Health for Glasgow, points out, " The value of the manufactured article depends sometimes on form and elasticity, which may be lost through heat; or on colour, which may be impaired. Every one knows that blankets and other woollen articles cannot be boiled without serious injury. Even the most cautious washing changes gradually the white, fleecy, new blanket into the yellow, dense, bare comparatively comfortless old one. With cottons and linens there is no trouble; they may be boiled with impunity. Wool, hair, and feathers are most troublesome. They all depend, for their value and utility, upon form and elasticity, which again depend, not only upon the hygrometric moisture, but upon the presence of certain fats. When we begin to deal with such articles, we find that we are involved in all the technical knowledge of several trade processes. . . . The practical result is constant friction in carrying out disinfection; temptation to public officials to scamp the work to avoid censure; constant private efforts to escape interference by concealment, or appeals to fictitious domestic processes; or on the part of the wealthy to resort to the general cleansing and renewing operations of the upholsterer and hair and feather cleaner."

If we wish to popularise disinfection, we must simplify the process as much as possible, having due regard to efficiency. It must never be forgotten that exposure to sunlight and fresh air constitutes one of the most effective means of disinfection that we possess, and it has the great advantages of involving no expense and but little trouble. Accordingly we find that in all regulations, intended to be observed by the public in general, great stress is laid upon the employment of those great natural disinfectants, fresh air and sunlight. Additional measures, easily carried out, should either precede or follow the exposure to air. Clothes, bedding, and all textile fabrics should be thoroughly washed with soap and hot water, left to soak for some hours in clean water, and then dried and exposed to air and sun for as many days as possible. Such articles as cannot be washed should be fumigated, in a manner presently to be described, either with chlorine or sulphurous acid, well shaken, beaten or brushed, and exposed freely for several days to sun and air. As a matter of course, all pillows, beds, mattresses, stuffed furniture, etc., should be cut open, the contents spread out and thoroughly fumigated. "Carpets are best fumigated on the floor, but should afterwards be removed to the open air and thoroughly beaten."

Dr. Russell states that, at Glasgow, simple washing has for many years been the sole method of disinfection applied by the sanitary authorities to all washable articles, and that the most careful investigation has failed to discover a single case of disease propagated by such materials. As a matter of course, every care is taken that the work is thoroughly done; the washing-house is constructed for the purpose, and provided with an ample supply of water and steam, and various mechanical appliances. All articles, with the exception of woollen fabrics, are purified by boiling or exposure to steam at a heat of 212°. Owing to the extreme softness of the water and the copiousness of the supply, Glasgow doubtless has many facilities for carrying out a system of disinfection which is, to a great extent, mechanical in its operation. Beating, shaking, and brushing are valuable auxiliaries in dealing with articles which cannot be properly washed.

For the disinfection of the air of rooms many substances are recommended and employed, but the way in which they are generally used causes them to act merely as deodorants. Even at the present day the fact is very incompletely realised that ventilation—that is, the continual admission of fresh air, coupled with the escape of air that has been contaminated—is the only effectual method of purifying the atmosphere of rooms occupied by patients suffering from infectious diseases. It is simply useless to place saucers containing chloride of lime, carbolic acid, or Condy's fluid in a contaminated atmosphere with the expectation that the germs floating about therein will be attracted, caught, and killed, like mice in a trap. The chlorine, doubtless, will readily diffuse itself throughout a room, and remove some offensive odours; but to act as a true disinfectant it must be so much concentrated, that the air thus charged with it would be quite irrespirable by human beings. It is, however, when used scientifically, the best disinfectant we possess for purifying the walls, etc., of an empty room. All the openings and chinks of such an apartment should be made as nearly air-tight as possible, and the evaporation of a large quantity of water in the room aids the action of the chlorine, which is easily generated by adding hydrochloric acid to bleaching powder.

If, however, large quantities are required, these are most readily and economically obtained by pouring two parts of sulphuric acid, of a specific gravity 1·535, over one part of bleaching powder, just enough water being then added to cause the latter to be covered. The gas may also be prepared in another way—viz., by mixing together common salt four parts, oxide of manganese three parts, sulphuric acid nine parts, and five parts of water. This process involves more expense and trouble than the method with bleaching powder. When chlorine is used for fumigating and disinfecting purposes, the vessels containing the mixture which evolves it should always be placed in the higher parts of the room, as it then descends on account of its density, and soon becomes mixed with the surrounding air. It must be remembered that chlorine, when combined with moisture, removes many vegetable colours from fabrics; it has little, if any, bleaching power when moisture is absent.

For *deodorising* purposes in sick-rooms and passages, a gas called "euchlorine" will be found very serviceable. It is produced when a few crystals of chlorate of potassium are dropped into a little hydrochloric acid. The mixture can be conveniently made in a small wide-mouthed bottle, which should be placed as near the ceiling as possible, so that the gas may descend into the room. Half an ounce of the strong acid will be found sufficient for several days; a few crystals of the chlorate, as many as can be taken between the finger and thumb, should be dropped in night and morning.

Bromine is even more powerful as a disinfectant than chlorine, but is not so convenient for use; both these agents are superior to sulphurous acid, which, however, possesses a considerable degree of efficacy, and is easily employed for disinfecting empty rooms. All openings and chinks should be closed as before, and a pound or more of sulphur should then be burnt in a brazier or other suitable vessel. The space to be disinfected should be kept saturated with the gas for a couple of hours or more. It must be remembered that sulphurous acid tarnishes and damages metals, and bleaches vegetable colours.

For the disinfection of walls and ceilings Professor Esmarch recommends that they should be rubbed down with bread, the pieces of which must be carefully collected and burnt. Experimenting in this way in the Berlin Hygienic Institute, he found that all germs were completely removed, and the rooms were rendered immediately habitable without danger. The rubbing is easily effected, and can be done at very little expense by untrained persons; it may also be used as a preliminary to disinfection by chlorine or sulphurous acid, both of which will penetrate into chinks and corners which cannot be reached by the hand.

Washing the surfaces by means of a spray containing disinfectants in solution is another efficacious method of purifying walls and ceilings, and the most potent substance which can be used in this manner is the perchloride of mercury or corrosive sublimate. The solution, which is highly poisonous to all forms of life, contains one part of the mineral in one thousand parts of water. A similar solution may be employed for the immersion of infected linen or clothing before washing; the articles should be allowed to remain in it for four hours at least.

Carbolic acid has been variously estimated as a disinfectant. For some years after it was first employed as a germicide it was considered to be the most efficacious substance of its class. Later on the preference was given to solutions of the perchloride of mercury; but since 1892, as the result of many experiments by Dr. Crookshank and others, the superiority of carbolic acid has again been demonstrated, and in surgical practice it is now regarded as the most powerful germicide. The question, however, may well be asked whether the highly diluted carbolic vapour used for purposes of aërial disinfection is not powerless to deal with an atmosphere saturated with the germs of infectious diseases. For the disinfection of liquids, a large amount of carbolic acid is required; the mixture should contain at least two per cent. by weight of the pure agent. Carbolic vapour will preserve for some months the freshness of a piece of meat suspended therein, and a very small quantity mixed with animal fluids keeps them fresh, and prevents all tendency to decomposition for an almost indefinite period. Milk can be thus preserved by the addition of one-fifth per cent. Carbolic acid will stop the progress of putrefactive changes, and, as Dr. J. A. Russell points out, "small quantities of this disinfectant, instead of destroying contagion, may actually preserve its activity, when otherwise it would have succumbed to the action of natural agencies. This danger may accompany the limited use of any disinfectant that has a 'pickling' or preservative action in small quantity." There is also another drawback connected with its use. Volatility is one of its properties, and "the acid may, for a time, deprive the contagion of its infective power, without permanently abolishing it, and the virulent properties may be regained whenever the acid has evaporated."

Condy's fluid—a solution of the permanganate of potassium—is much employed for general purposes of disinfection and deodorisation. It is a very efficacious deodorant of fluid matters, and has the advantage of being non-poisonous; but to act as a real disinfectant—that is, to destroy contagious germs or abolish their power of reproduction—it must be used in very large quantities, and is therefore expensive. It is admirably adapted for deodorising offensive matters in the sick-room, and to these it should be added until its colour remains. It is likewise well adapted for pouring down drains and sinks, and a supply of it should be kept in every house. Ozone may be prepared from it by adding three parts of strong sulphuric acid to two parts of the salt dissolved in water; and this, like the permanganate itself, oxidises organic matter and thus destroys offensive emanations, and, moreover, being gaseous, will diffuse itself through the air, whereas the permanganate is non-volatile. Ozone is also evolved from terebene, which is a very effective and pleasant deodorant when used with a spray apparatus.

For the disinfection of sinks, drains, etc., the permanganate has already been advised; carbolic acid and the chloride of zinc (Burnett's solution) are also efficacious. A perchloride of mercury solution, eight grains to a gallon, is an extremely powerful disinfectant; but the mercury is precipitated when brought into contact with copper, lead, and tin, and it renders leaden pipes very brittle. The stronger acids are liable to objections of the same character.

Some of the statements made in preceding paragraphs will now be summarised, so as to indicate the methods of carrying out disinfection under the various circumstances in which it is required.

A patient suffering from a contagious disease

must be prevented from becoming a source of danger to the healthy. Infective matters are being constantly given off from his body, and every care must be taken to prevent these from being conveyed to others by attendants, by clothes, bed-linen, etc., or through discharges of all kinds. Free ventilation into the open air, through windows, provides for the escape of noxious emanations, which are rendered harmless by dilution. After recovery, the patient, nurses, all clothes, the sick-room and its furniture must be thoroughly disinfected.

The measures best calculated to ensure these objects are as follows :—

1. The patient must be isolated in a separate room, at the top of the house, if possible. All unnecessary articles of furniture, woollen materials especially, must be removed from the room before the patient is placed in it. Carpets and woollen curtains are favourite resting-places of morbid germs, and are disinfected and cleansed with difficulty. All drawers, cupboards, etc., should be emptied. Staircase windows should be kept open night and day, so as thoroughly to ventilate the house. The door of the patient's room must

be kept closed as much as possible, and outside should be suspended a cloth saturated with a solution of carbolic acid, chloride of zinc, or with dilute Condy's fluid. This should never be allowed to become dry. The windows in the room must be kept open whenever circumstances will permit, and except in hot weather a fire should be kept burning. The destruction of unpleasant odours is best effected by euchlorine (see pages 254 *et sqq.*). The patient's attendants should not visit other parts of the house, and it will be an advantage in most cases to select persons who have already had the disease. The medical attendant will adopt all necessary precautions to prevent himself from becoming a carrier of contagion. With regard to the residents in the house, there is no risk in allowing them to continue their ordinary avocations, and to leave the premises as usual, provided that the patient is kept properly isolated, and plenty of fresh air is allowed to circulate in the house. Vessels, cups, and plates used for feeding the patient should be kept upstairs, and articles of food or drink left by the patient should be destroyed.

2. All the discharges from the patient should be disinfected before being carried downstairs. If they are to be thrown into the drains, the best disinfectants are carbolic acid, chloride of zinc, and permanganate of potassium. These should be freely employed; small quantities are utterly useless. Whenever the discharges can be buried deep in earth (an excellent method of disposing of them) quicklime should be added in excess, or a strong solution of perchloride of mercury (four grains to a pint of water) should be mixed with them. In country places where fuel is readily procurable, burning the discharges in the open air is an excellent way of destroying contagious germs.

3. For disinfecting the sheets and body-linen used by the patient, the methods already described must be carefully employed (see page 252). As soon as the clothes are removed from the patient or his bed, they should be placed in a wooden tub containing a solution of perchloride of mercury (two grains to a pint). After remaining for twelve hours, they may be removed, rinsed in clean water, and sent to be washed.

4. When the patient is convalescent, he should be carefully washed with hot water and carbolic or thymol soap; and, as soon as he is able to bear them, a few warm baths will have a very beneficial effect. His hair should be thoroughly cleansed, and he should be dressed in clothes which have not been in his room, and taken into another apartment. The attendants should adopt similar precautions with regard to washing, change of clothes, etc.

5. The room, when vacated by the patient, should be thoroughly cleansed and disinfected. All movable articles should be taken away, washed, exposed to heat, and then to air and sunlight. Especial care is necessary in dealing with bedding, wool, and feathers. Leather and other articles which would be destroyed or greatly damaged by heat should be sponged with carbolic acid diluted with forty parts of water. With regard to the room itself, the best means of disinfecting it have been already described (see pages 251 *et sqq.*). Chlorine and sulphurous acid are the best gaseous disinfectants, and are easily generated. The floor should be thoroughly scrubbed, the ceiling

scraped and whitewashed, the walls repapered or rubbed over with bread, and the paint washed with carbolic soap. It is impossible to take too much pains in carrying out these measures of disinfection. After they are completed, the windows and door of the room should be left open night and day for a fortnight at least before the room is again occupied.

It is quite certain that the germs of some infectious diseases, notably cholera and typhoid fever, are conveyed into the human body through the medium of drinking-water. When compelled to make use of water of a suspicious class, filtration and boiling constitute the most reliable methods of purification. Spongy iron is, upon the whole, the most efficacious filtering material. The water, especially if passed through sand afterwards, comes out quite clear and pure, and may be kept for a long time without showing any signs of the production of living organisms. The Chamberland-Pasteur filter effectually strains off all organisms and their spores; but it has little or no effect upon dissolved constituents. Charcoal filters, on the other hand, certainly sometimes allow spores or germs to pass through unchanged, and when they are employed, boiling should always be superadded. It is not sufficient to bring the water once to the boiling-point; in order to be efficacious, repeated boilings are necessary, for the reasons given in a preceding paragraph. Milk of a suspicious character should always be thus thoroughly boiled. Travellers on the Continent do well to provide themselves with small portable filters, now easily procurable, for in many places the drinking-water is highly charged with impurities. It is satisfactory to know that the tannin contained in tea is a purifying agent of some value as regards organic matter present in water.

In order to complete this sketch of the present state of our knowledge with regard to infection, and of the best methods of preventing the spread of infectious diseases, it seems desirable to give a short account of the public arrangements having the latter object for their aim. In the metropolis every vestry and district board must appoint one or more legally qualified medical practitioners of skill and experience as officers of health. The duties of such officers are, among others, to ascertain the existence of diseases, more especially epidemics, and to point out the best means of checking or preventing their spread. Under the Public Health Act, 1875, the whole of England, with the exception of the metropolis, is divided into sanitary districts, placed under the charge of certain authorities, who must appoint, from time to time, a medical officer of health, whose duties have been clearly defined by the Local Government Board. We have, therefore, at the present time, in every part of the country, highly-trained medical officers of health, performing duties of a manifold character, having for their objects the prevention of the breaking-out and spread of disease, and the improvement of the general health of the public at large. It is not too much to say that the efficient performance of these duties, aided by the co-operation of those most nearly concerned, cannot fail to lessen the number of cases of infectious disease, and might, indeed, in time, cause some of these affections to disappear from the Registrar-General's returns. One of these duties is described in the following regulation: "On receiving information of the outbreak of a contagious, infectious, or epidemic disease, the medical officer shall visit the spot, inquire into the causes and circumstances of the outbreak, advise as to measures for preventing the extension of the disease, and assist in executing the same."

Up to 1889 Parliament had dealt with the subject of the notification of infectious diseases in a very imperfect and unsatisfactory manner. It had promulgated no general law applicable to all communities; but had simply permitted regulations on the subject to be inserted in a few local Bills. In most places it was no one's business to report the existence of cases of infectious disease to the sanitary authorities; in a few localities, only the medical attendant was charged with this duty; and in others the householder was likewise bound to make a report. The differences have to a large extent been abolished by the Act passed in 1889, which charges both the medical attendant and the head of the family to which the patient belongs (or some other person connected with him), as soon as they become aware that the case is one to which the Act applies, to send a certificate, giving certain necessary particulars, to the medical officer of health. Failure to give such notice renders the persons liable to a fine not exceeding forty shillings; and the diseases to which the Act applies are, in all places, small-pox, cholera, diphtheria, membranous croup, erysipelas, scarlatina (scarlet fever), and the fevers known by any of the following names: typhus, typhoid, enteric, relapsing, continued or puerperal.

The sanitary authority of any district may, with the consent of the Local Government Board, add any other infectious disease to the above category; but the adoption of the Act is nowhere compulsory, though in June of last year it was in force among twenty-seven out of twenty-nine millions of people in England and Wales. It would seem that the time has come when the Act should be enforced by statute in every district of the country: those districts which neglect to do all in their power to check the spread of disease should not be allowed to endanger neighbouring districts.

I must not bring this essay to a conclusion without stating that there are many disinfectants now offered to the public, but which regard to space and the purpose I had in view have prevented me from describing. I have thought it best to confine my remarks to such disinfectants as are really efficacious, and to point out the advantages and drawbacks connected with their use. With respect to many so-called "disinfectants," it is sufficient to say that their power has been absurdly over-estimated. It cannot be too strongly insisted upon that deodorisation is by no means equivalent to disinfection. My object has been to indicate in the first place what in the present state of our knowledge seems to be the true theory as to the causation of infectious diseases, and to show how obstacles are presented to more rapid scientific progress by the extreme minuteness of the organisms with which we have to deal. With regard to disinfection, I have striven to prove how entirely it must depend for its success on the specific action exercised upon the disease-germs by the means employed. The realisation of this necessary relation cannot fail to dispel many a fond belief with regard to disinfectants; but it will leave us with a more intelligent and useful appreciation of their true properties, and, by revealing how far we still are from the goal of complete knowledge, may even stimulate the investigator to explore paths of science which are yet unknown. Virgil says, "Felix qui potuit rerum cognoscere causas," and to nothing is this aphorism more applicable than to a knowledge of those agencies which produce infectious diseases.

XI.

THE LONDON WATER SUPPLY.

THE importance of a sufficient supply of wholesome water for domestic purposes is at the present day admitted by all who have paid any attention to the subject. Water is a necessity of life, second only to the air we breathe. It or its elements form about four-fifths of the human body, and without its assistance no function can be discharged. It is a necessary constituent of all food, and is of itself the most valuable of the many articles which come under this denomination. Life can be supported for days and even for weeks upon water alone, and its admixture with so-called solid foods is a necessary condition of their being utilised by the animal system. Although some substances resist its action as a solvent, its power in this respect is much more extensive than that of any other fluid.

CONTAMINATION OF SOURCES.

Water has other valuable properties. It is the most effective and convenient agent for cleansing the surface of our bodies, our clothes, furniture, and dwellings, and the soil itself; and when it descends in the form of rain, it cleanses the air by washing the impurities out of it. Its physical properties and the ease with which it can be set in motion render it the most convenient channel for the removal of many waste and effete materials, and for their conveyance to places suitable for their disposal, and it is especially this use of water which has led to so many difficulties and dangers in connection with its supply to large communities. Abundance of wholesome water is almost everywhere obtainable, but unfortunately its sources and the streams in which it flows are too often contaminated by the admixture of filthy and noxious matters. Such contamination is not only repulsive to all ideas of cleanliness, but it includes many great dangers, for not a few epidemics of fatal diseases have been caused by the germs of such disorders having gained access to the water. It is now pretty generally known that any sudden outbreak of disease in an epidemic form is almost certainly attributable to the water supply, that is, to something which has passed into the water, and has been swallowed by the sufferers.

In primitive communities and in sparsely scattered populations there is seldom much difficulty in obtaining a supply of water. Wells are sunk; and if these are properly protected from contamination, the supply, as a general rule, is abundant and wholesome. In Eastern countries, such as India, in which water is the only fluid drunk by the natives, the popular taste becomes so far educated as to be able to distinguish good water from bad; it is generally safe to use water from those wells that are the most frequented. Palatable water is, however, not necessarily pure water, and well water is peculiarly liable to contamination, not only from matters thrown or falling into it, but from noxious substances which soak through the surrounding soil.

When, however, extensive communities inhabiting large cities have to be supplied with water, the problem is one of a very different character. To obtain sufficient water of any kind must often be difficult; to obtain wholesome water may be almost, if not quite, impossible. A supply cannot be obtained on the spot; if thousands of wells were sunk in a large city, some would yield bad water, all would be liable to contamination, and the supply would eventually prove insufficient. Water must therefore be brought from a distance, and whenever large towns are in the vicinity of rivers, the most natural course to pursue is to take the water thus brought within reach by natural agencies. River water, free from admixture with extraneous matters, is generally of excellent quality. Many rivers begin in clear mountain streams of pure water, and receive accessions to their volume, not only from tributary streams, but from the ground—water which, having fallen as rain on higher ground, has sunk in, to reappear in sandy or gravelly regions at lower levels in the form of springs. If rivers were simply channels for the passage of water, if no effete and waste materials were allowed to pass into them, we should hear very little about the difficulties of supplying water to the majority of large cities. Up to quite recent times, rivers have been regarded as the most convenient receptacles for sewage and waste matters of all kinds, and even modern legislation against such pollution has not achieved the desired object, though considerable improvement has been effected. It may be laid down as a general rule that no stream ought to be used both as a source of supply and as a carrier of waste and excrementitious materials.

In applying this rule, however, to the case of large cities, and especially to that of our own metropolis, we are confronted with several facts of a very remarkable character. Were not the results of experience constantly before us, to provide five millions of human beings with a never-failing supply of water would probably be regarded as an impossibility, and it is still difficult to realise the magnitude of the operations by which the supply is effected. The simple fact is, that eight large water companies supply one hundred and fifty-four million gallons daily to a population amounting in the aggregate to nearly five-and-a-half millions, the consumption being at the rate of twenty-eight gallons a head, and nearly half of the total quantity supplied being taken from the Thames. More than one-third comes from the Lea, while the remainder is supplied from springs and wells. It follows, therefore, that five-sixths of the total quantity of water supplied to the metropolis is derived from sources condemned by the rule laid down in the previous paragraph.

The eight water companies are authorised to obtain their supply from the following sources:—Five of them—viz., the Southwark and Vauxhall, the West Middlesex, the Grand Junction, the Lambeth and the Chelsea companies take water from the Thames at Hampton, Molesey, and Ditton, the maximum quantity allowed in twenty-four hours being one hundred and twenty millions of gallons. The East London Company gets its supply from the River Lea, at Chingford, and is also allowed to take, when necessary, as much as ten millions of gallons daily from the Thames at Sunbury. The New River Company takes water from the Lea, near Ware, the spring at Chadwell, and from thirteen chalk wells in the Lea valley. The Kent Waterworks Company obtains its supply from the chalk wells between Deptford and Crayford.

All these companies contract to collect water

from intakes, or certain defined spots where it is obtainable, to store it in proper reservoirs, filter it, bring it into the streets, maintain it under a given pressure, and convey it into the private service pipes provided at the expense of the house owner or the consumer. The companies' engagements are completed when the water is brought, in a wholesome and pure condition, to the premises of the consumer as required by the "Metropolis Water Act, 1871," and when provision is made for a regular supply. They are not responsible for anything which may happen to the water inside the premises supplied. It may be kept in filthy cisterns, it may absorb gases from drains or cesspools, and may become absolutely poisonous; but for such contamination, and for the state of the pipes within the house, the builder or householder is responsible. What is perhaps still more important, because less generally known, the water companies are not responsible for much of the deterioration of quality at the intakes, from the neglect of local public authorities, such as river conservators and others, who have allowed increasing quantities of sewage or refuse matter to be discharged into the river above the points whence the supplies are taken for public consumption.

Such, then, are the present arrangements for supplying London and its five and-a-half millions of inhabitants with water. They have been completed at a cost of over fourteen millions sterling, and since the passing of the "Metropolis Water Act, 1871," the companies have incurred and undertaken an expenditure amounting to upwards of four millions for the improvement of the water supply, both in quantity and quality, for extending the capacity of their reservoirs, and increasing the areas of filtration, as well as for providing for the requirements of a constant supply. In order that the consumers' interests should be duly protected, the "Metropolis Water Act" of 1871 provided for the appointment of a water examiner, being a competent and impartial person, who should from time to time examine the water supplied by the companies, to ascertain whether they had complied with the requirements of Section 4 of the "Metropolis Water Act, 1852," which orders that every company shall effectually filter all water supplied by them within the metropolis for domestic use before the same shall pass into the pipes for distribution. The filtration of water taken from the Thames and Lea is effected by the water companies in the following manner.

The water is received into subsidiary reservoirs, and there stored for some days, during which a large proportion of the suspended matter gradually subsides, when the water is drawn off into the filter-beds. These large reservoirs have another advantage; they enable the companies to increase their storage during fair weather, and to discontinue the collection during temporary floods. In 1877 the total storage of the seven companies was 1,041 millions of gallons; in 1888, 1,290 millions, or about nine days' supply. The water supplied by the Kent Company, being taken from deep wells in the chalk, does not require filtering.

The filtering-beds are composed of gravel and sand, the depth of the materials thus employed varying from three-and-a-half to seven feet (see report by Water Examiner for Nov. 1888). The upper layer of about two feet is composed of sand, the remainder is made up of gravel. Sometimes a layer of shells is placed between the sand and gravel, gradually increasing in coarseness. The pressure of the water in these filters is not great, the depth is never more than two feet, and it is found that sixty gallons pass through each square foot in twenty-four hours. The filtering-beds are cleansed and replenished with fresh sand from time to time. The action of the sand is mainly of a mechanical nature; it certainly removes suspended matter, both organic and mineral, and it appears to retain about 5 per cent. of the dissolved constituents; and the power of such a filter in arresting organisms is considerable when the sand is fresh, but it ceases after a time. Dr. R. Koch, however, states that the reduction in the number of organisms is due to the film of mud which gradually forms on the surface of sand-filters, and which mechanically retains the organisms in the same manner as a Pasteur filter, in which the water is forced through unglazed biscuit ware. If this statement be correct, it must be regarded as unfortunate that the film has to be scraped off periodically, in order to allow of the percolation of the water through the filter. The removal of the film takes place about once a month; and as Dr. Koch states that a fortnight is required before it acts as a good filtering medium, as against organisms, it is clear that in our waterworks there must always be several filter-beds which offer but a slight obstacle to the passage of microphytes, which may have gained access to the water. Against this drawback, however, is to be set the fact, already alluded to, that fine white sand, well washed, arrests the passage of a considerable proportion of organisms. It does not afford complete protection, for it was shown at Lausen, in Switzerland, that water containing typhoid germs, after having been subjected to sand-filtration, infected the population of a village and destroyed many lives. Ferruginous green-sand and spongy iron are still more efficient in this respect (see Dr. Frankland's Report on the use of spongy iron in the filter-beds of the Antwerp water-works). The duties of the water examiner are of a multifarious character. He inspects the filter-beds and reservoirs, and examines the quality of the water at the intakes and after filtration. He furnishes monthly and annual reports, giving complete and exact information with regard to the water supplied, including such points as its source, total volume, average daily supply, state of filtration, condition of samples, etc. He furnishes reports on the composition and quality of daily samples of the water, based on analyses made for the companies by analysts of their own appointment, and by an analyst chosen by the Government; and lastly a report of results of the bacteriological examination of the metropolitan water supply made by Dr. Percy Frankland.

From the foregoing account of the precautions taken to insure that the water when delivered to the consumer shall be as pure as circumstances will permit, it is obvious that no charge of neglect can be sustained against the companies or those who control their operations. With regard to the companies, it is universally admitted that they have always been in advance of public opinion on improvements in the water supply; not only do they fulfil their contracts, but they do not limit themselves to a bare compliance with the provisions of Acts of Parliament, they frequently adopt measures for the general improvement of the supplies, and exhibit proofs of their anxiety to discharge the duties of their position towards the public. It cannot be said that the inhabitants of London are dissatisfied with the water supplied to them. Possibly their satisfaction may be the result of ignorance or indifference; but there can be no doubt as to its widespread existence. With regard, however, to the source of supply and the consequent quality of the water, very conflicting opinions are held by men who deserve to be regarded as competent authorities. If we are to believe Dr. Frankland and those who think with him, there may be water everywhere in London, but there is not a drop fit to drink, except that which is supplied from the chalk wells in Kent. Other able chemists agree with Dr. Tidy in declaring that the London water is excellent, and that no better sources of supply can be found for the metropolis, considering all the facts of the case, than the rivers Thames and Lea. It will be well to examine briefly the evidence adduced in support of these two contradictory opinions. There is, however, a preliminary question which must not be passed over: every one wishes to secure pure water, but what is the standard of purity? Now *pure* water, using the adjective in the strict sense, is not obtainable outside the chemist's laboratory, and much care is required for its preparation. It is obtained by distilling ordinary good water, and the product has to be tested in various ways in order to determine that it has received no contamination from the vessels employed in the process. If no mineral matters are discoverable, and if on evaporation the water leaves "scarcely a visible residue," it may be regarded as pure. Next to distilled water comes rain water, caught in clean vessels, on mountains or large plains far from human habitations and after some hours of rain. It is almost needless to say that water up to this standard of purity is not to be found in the purest springs or rivers. These are supplied by rain which falls on the earth, charged with many impurities washed out of the atmosphere, and capable of dissolving many materials on and beneath the earth's surface. Lime and magnesia are universally present in the soil, and various organic matters offer themselves for solution. As water sinks through the earth, new materials are taken up; others previously dissolved or suspended in the fluid are often retained. Hence spring water contains the results of solution modified by filtration. River water, containing as it does much rain water that has fallen on the earth, is apt to vary greatly in composition, and often contains much organic matter washed off the surface by the rain.

Water, whether from river or spring, to be regarded as wholesome, must be perfectly clear, free from odour, tasteless, and cold. It must also contain more or less air and carbonic acid (otherwise it will taste flat); and it must be soft, through the absence of undue amounts of lime and magnesia. Its solid constituents should not be much more than ten grains in a gallon, except in the case of water from chalk wells, where that proportion may be much exceeded. With regard to the organic matter —an all-important question—if water from the chalk springs of the Kent Company be taken as a standard, there should not be more than one-tenth of a grain in a gallon. It is very difficult to distinguish between dissolved organic matter derived from vegetable substances and that of animal origin. Elaborate chemical processes are required, and the chances of error are considerable. Some information may be obtained by examining the sediment with the microscope, and from a consideration of the source of the water and the various matters dissolved therein. Bacteria of all kinds, fungi, remains of animal structures, eggs of parasites, etc., must be absent. Infusorial animalcules of various kinds and diatoms are often seen in well waters, and do not indicate any serious impurity. To make an exhaustive examination of a given sample of water requires considerable skill, but its wholesomeness or otherwise can generally be decided without much difficulty. It is perhaps necessary to mention the fact that the taste of water is a very uncertain indication of its purity. If anything objectionable be detected by the tongue, the water must be rejected; but dissolved organic matter is often tasteless, and the sense of taste is of little use in discovering many dissolved mineral substances. Thus common salt is recognised by the tongue only when a gallon of water contains as much as seventy grains. On the other hand, very small quantities of iron communicate a peculiar flavour to the water; one-fifth of a grain per gallon can be thus discovered. It is well to warm water before tasting it; cold is always grateful to the tongue, and prevents many unpleasant flavours from being noticed.

Having thus briefly alluded to the characteristics of wholesome water, I proceed to inquire whether the water supplied to the metropolis can be included in this category. It cannot be denied that a considerable amount of sewage and refuse matter enters the Thames above the spots at which the water is taken by the various companies. It has, indeed, been stated that the sewage from a population estimated at more than half a million is thus disposed of, and that therefore the source of supply is contaminated to such a degree as absolutely to condemn the water even if filtered through sand in the best possible way. It must be remembered that the "Rivers Pollution Act" forbids the discharge in their entirety of sewage matters into rivers. The most common methods of dealing with sewage are to allow the solid parts to subside or to precipitate the greater portion by means of chemical substances, and then to make provision for the liquid to pass over or through land and thence into a stream. The sewer water is to some extent purified, but its standard of purity has not as yet been fixed. Besides this source of contamination, the result of floods must be taken into account. The cultivated ground near the banks of the upper Thames is often under water, and much organic matter from manure, decaying vegetables, etc., must be washed into the river as the floods subside. Another source of impurity—viz., the refuse from house-boats and from the floating population—must also be borne in mind. To express numerically the condition of the Thames water, it may be assumed that from four to five hundred millions of gallons pass daily over Teddington Lock, and that twenty million gallons of dilute sewage have been mixed with it. The potential impurity may be described as fluctuating between 2 and 4 per cent.

It is all-important to determine as accurately as possible whether this degree of impurity represents a fixed quantity, or whether it is lessened as the water flows on. Much turns upon the answer given to this question; as usual, very conflicting evidence is given by experts, but an unbiassed examination would appear to show that rivers with a flow of a few miles possess considerable power of transforming hurtful organic impurities into harmless products. The change is effected by three principal agencies. (1) The suspended organic matters subside; they are forcibly carried to the bottom by the admixture of the impure water with suspended mineral matters. (2) Fish act as scavengers, and it must be remembered that their presence in water indicates a certain degree of purity. (3) The most potent purifying agent is oxygen, derived in part from the air and in part from the plant life with which rivers abound. The oxygen derived from the latter source being set free in the water, is the more powerful agent in producing the change. The weeds of a river bed into which sewage passes absorb a large amount of organic matter and of chlorides, and are valuable purifiers of the water.

Dr. Frankland admits that some purifying

action may occur in the course of the flow of a river, but contends that it is so small as to be practically useless. He considers that if the water of a river be once contaminated with ever so small a proportion of sewage matters, no river in England is long enough to bring about, by oxidation or otherwise, such a removal of the organic impurities as to render the water wholesome and fit for domestic use. He cites the case of the river Irwell, which, after passing Manchester, runs eleven miles to its junction with the Mersey without further material pollution, and falls over six weirs; yet the purification by oxidation is trifling. Dr. Tidy, on the other hand, asserts that if sewage be discharged into a river and mixed with at least twenty times its volume of pure water, after a moderately rapid flow of a few miles, the whole of the impurities will disappear as a result of oxidation and other agencies, and the water will be restored to its original state of purity. The late Dr. Parkes—an authority second to none on such a subject—was inclined to attribute much influence to oxidation, and several facts strongly support this view. The case of the river Tees deserves to be mentioned; this river receives the sewage of Barnard Castle, containing four thousand inhabitants, and of several villages, and likewise the refuse from dyeworks and fellmongers. It flows on for sixteen miles to Darlington, where the water companies supplying that town, Stockton, and Middlesbrough obtain their water. It is somewhat remarkable that Dr. Frankland has reported this water to be "of unimpeachable quality, as clear and bright (after filtration), and nearly as palatable, as deep well or spring water." Here, surely, there is no evidence of previous sewage contamination.

Another remarkable instance of the purification of water as a result of free exposure to the air was furnished by Mr. A. le Grand, in a communication to the Society of Arts. He was well acquainted with the water of a river known to be more or less polluted, and of which samples were sent to analysts from time to time. On one occasion the water as drawn from the river was forced up into the air in a jet, and the spray which fell was collected and sent to the analyst. So great was the change in the direction of purity that the analyst, until assured by competent authority, was sceptical as to the real source of the water. These instances seem to prove that exposure to air purifies water contaminated with organic matter. Such exposure must, however, be complete and continuous. It is not contended that well water conveyed in pipes can be thus improved, though this admission is sometimes cited by the opponents of the oxidation theory in support of their view. About eighteen years ago the chalk wells at Caterham became polluted by a workman suffering from typhoid fever, and the result was that many persons in Redhill who drank the water were attacked by the disease. Now, the distance between these two places is about seven miles, and it is not fair to assume that, because the typhoid poison was capable of being conveyed that distance in closed pipes, its effects would have been the same had it passed into a river and been swallowed after a flow of some miles.

If it were true that no improvement, whether by oxidation or otherwise, takes place in river water during its flow, and if sewage-matter, even in very small amount, could not possibly be excluded, it would be absolutely necessary to seek other sources of supply. Dr. Frankland's opinion is that we ought to have two systems of water supply in London: the first ought to give us good water fit for dietetic purposes; the second, water for manufacturing and trading purposes, flushing sewers, watering streets, and extinguishing fires. It would not, however, be desirable to introduce two kinds of water into houses, for most servants, not to speak of other persons, would go to the nearest tap, whatever the quality of the water. Only the pure water should be introduced in houses, and the use of meters should be compulsory, so as to prevent waste. Dr. Frankland thinks that it is quite unnecessary to continue to supply some thirty gallons per head, as is done in London, and that ten gallons would be sufficient. He would obtain this pure water from springs or deep wells, and convey it to the consumer without previous admixture of sewage and other impurities. Such wells can be found in the Thames Valley, for it is a well-known fact that in times of long drought the Thames is supplied exclusively from springs almost all coming from the chalk and the oolite. It certainly seems unnecessary to take enormous pains to purify water which is used only for watering streets and other outdoor purposes. Even Thames water taken at London Bridge, if a few days were allowed for the subsidence of the coarser impurities, would be sufficiently pure for such uses. With regard to the average supply to each individual, twenty-eight gallons daily is probably excessive. There is doubtless much waste from carelessness and bad taps, but it is desirable that any error in the quantity supplied should be on the side of excess. Habits of cleanliness are not too common, and nothing should be done that would tend to make them less popular, or to furnish excuses for negligence. Waste of water should, however, be checked in every possible way. Dr. Parkes estimated that for personal and domestic use, without baths, twelve gallons per head daily should be given as a minimum supply, and that with baths and perfect cleanliness sixteen gallons should be allowed. Water for necessary sanitary purposes is not included in this estimate, and it must be remembered that even a small general bath (4 feet long and 1 foot 9 inches wide) for an adult will require from thirty to forty gallons.

If the Thames is to be superseded or supplemented as a source of water supply in the manner suggested by Dr. Frankland, it would be necessary to inquire into the capacity of springs and wells to afford the requisite *quantity* of water. It is, perhaps, too readily assumed that no grounds for fear would exist with regard to the *quality*. Water from the best chalk wells is clear, transparent, and bright; it is well aerated, and free from dead organic matter, and contains comparatively few organisms. Its hardness is its only drawback, and this depends upon the presence of an excessive amount of chalk, held in solution by carbonic acid gas. It may be softened by adding lime, with which the carbonic acid unites; the chalk is then thrown down and withdrawn from the water. It must never be forgotten that well water may be, and often is, highly impure, and this is notoriously the case with shallow wells in porous soils. A well drains an extent of ground around it nearly in the shape of an inverted cone, and the water which soaks in from the soil is often very impure. The area drained must depend upon the soil: Dr. Parkes states that the distance ranges from fifteen to one hundred and sixty times the depression of the water in the well. The deepest (non-Artesian) well will drain a cone, in a loose soil of chalk or sand, of about half a mile in radius. All water from deep wells must come from the surface, and, as pointed out by Professor Bischof, the question as to how far it is purified in passing from the surface of the soil to the bottom of a well is a very important one. It is often assumed that the water has filtered through hundreds of feet of solid rock, but it is certain that much water often passes directly through fissures, and does not gradually find its way through minute interstices. Thus, even deep wells have been known to contain seeds, stems, and roots of certain marsh plants, and even small fishes and shells. These deep wells are often fed by leaky beds of rivers, and the danger of contaminating them is increased in proportion to the amount withdrawn by the pumping and lowering of the ground water. Well water often contains germs, and the chemical purification may be only an increase of that performed by the ordinary sand-filter. All these points require to be considered in the examination of any projects for supplying large communities with water from wells and springs.

Admitting the comparative purity of deep well water, it must not be forgotten that the opinions of experts differ considerably as to the *quantity* obtainable from these sources. If we may judge from experience—probably the safest guide in the question before us—not a few deep wells would sooner or later become exhausted if large supplies of water were drawn from them. It must not be supposed that the water passing into these wells is contained in huge reservoirs which could be drawn upon *ad infinitum*. Between the months of May and November in ordinary years but little water is received into the chalk area, and the quantity becomes gradually diminished. The replenishment depends on the winter rainfall, the quantity of which influences the next year's supply. When the first Artesian well was sunk in the chalk under London the water rose freely above the surface of the ground; its level is now 60 or 70 feet below it. When the

Hanwell Asylum well was first bored, and for some time afterwards, the water rose 18 feet; at the present day it has to be pumped up. A similar and still more striking example is afforded by the well at Richmond. When this was first sunk, thirty years ago, water rushed up and overflowed; now it has sunk 120 feet. These instances prove that there is no permanent storage of water, and that the supply is likely to be exhausted. There is another difficulty, though a less serious one, connected with obtaining a large supply from wells. Mr. Baldwin Latham has pointed out that water cannot be taken from water-bearing strata by means of a well without diminishing the quantity which would otherwise flow out by natural streams; hence manufacturers with works on the banks of streams might find their industries crippled by withdrawal of the water upon the supply of which they depend.

Apart from the natural objections against drinking water in any way contaminated with sewage matter, there is the risk of the propagation of serious diseases, the germs of which passing with the discharges into water are afterwards swallowed. The evidence that typhoid fever and cholera may be thus spread is quite convincing, and there is much probability that other disorders are disseminated in a similar manner, though the connection between them and impurity of water cannot always be clearly demonstrated. Typhoid fever has again and again been shown to be propagated through the medium of water; the Caterham epidemic, already alluded to, is a case in point. Ordinary sewage matter may produce diarrhœa even of a serious character, but for the production of typhoid the specific germ must be present. The truth of this statement is shown by those instances collected by Dr. W. Budd and others, in which persons had for years been drinking water contaminated with ordinary sewage, but no cases of typhoid had occurred until a sufferer from the disease came into the place, and the discharges from this patient were washed into the stream from which the water supply was obtained. The evidence that cholera may be propagated through the medium of the water supply is equally strong. Dr. Parkes has collected many instances, and remarks that each successive example adds more and more weight to those previously observed, until, from the mere accumulation of cases, the cogency of the argument becomes irresistible. It may be added that in all probability the continuous use of water containing much organic matter lowers the resisting powers of the body, and renders it a more favourable nidus for the germs of specific disease.

The diseases just referred to are supposed to be caused by the presence of living organisms termed bacteria, microphytes, or more generally disease-germs. The discovery and study of these organisms date from a comparatively recent period; an enormous amount of attention has been devoted to them, but so far with only negative results as regards their differentiation, with comparatively few exceptions. High powers of the microscope are required for their detection, and it is often impossible to say whether those present in a given specimen of water are similar to others taken from another source. It would appear, moreover, that these organisms or their germs may exist in water and yet may be beyond detection by the highest powers of the microscope. When their presence is suspected, the test by " cultivation," as it is termed, is now employed. A fluid containing sugar, tartrate of ammonium, burnt yeast ash and water is found to be an excellent breeding-ground. A little of this fluid is boiled in a test-tube, which has previously been exposed to great heat, a few drops of the water are added, and the mouth of the tube is closed with cotton wool. If bacteria or their germs exist in the water, in a few days the liquid becomes milky from the presence of countless organisms. Inasmuch, however, as bacteria are to be found in the purest kinds of natural water, this test is not a positive indication of the quality of any given sample. It is, however, useful when taken in connection with other methods; and if the water rapidly becomes opalescent, the organisms may be assumed to be comparatively abundant.

The bacteriological examination of the metropolitan water supply is now regularly conducted by Dr. Percy Frankland, and the results are published in the monthly report. A small, measured portion of the water is mixed with gelatine and other nutritive media spread on glass plates and set aside in a cultivating apparatus. In a few days so-called " colonies " of minute organisms will be discoverable. These can be counted with the aid of the microscope, and are described as so many in a given cubic space. The significance of the different forms has not yet been determined, and there is no test which will distinguish those which are the germs of disease from those which are harmless. Dr. Bischof has pointed out a curious fact in connection with the development of bacteria. If samples of unfiltered water be stored in flasks, the organisms undergo no increase, but soon diminish in numbers. If filtered water be stored, the organisms increase enormously, perhaps because the filtration has removed some which would prevent the development of others. Thus the Kent chalk water contains but very few organisms; if it be bottled and kept in a warm place for a few days, millions make their appearance. If unfiltered river water were thus treated, the result would be of an entirely opposite character.

It is obvious that myriads of bacteria are constantly finding their way into the water of the Thames; they are known to possess great vitality and to be capable of resisting the action of many chemical agents. They are, however, destroyed by very slight differences of acidity and by changes of composition in the fluid. Fortunately, the composition of the Thames water undergoes very frequent alterations, and it varies in different places. Wholesale destruction of organisms is the probable result, and their removal from water is certainly effected by repeated and thorough filtration. Dr. Percy Frankland stated that their average reduction as a result of the treatment in the reservoirs of the companies amounted in 1877 to 96·7 per cent. If this be correct it is satisfactory to know that the removal of organisms by filtration can be readily accomplished, and it follows that the propagation of diseases through the medium of the Thames water is, under present arrangements, extremely improbable. It might, indeed, be rendered impossible, if ordinary care were taken by householders still further to purify the water supplied to them. Drinking-water should never be taken from cisterns, and a filter should find a place in every house, for there is no difficulty in obtaining an efficient apparatus. A preliminary caution is necessary: a filter which cannot be cleaned, and in which there is no provision for renewing the materials, is fraught with danger. So called "self-cleaning filters requiring no attention" should be carefully shunned; for if filters act effectually, they must sooner or later contain a large quantity of objectionable matters, some of which will be communicated to the water intended to be purified. Various materials are used in domestic filters, the principal being animal charcoal, spongy iron, and magnetic oxide of iron. All these materials are more or less efficient; but the spongy iron appears to be the most potent purifying agent at present available. In the Sixth Report of the Rivers Pollution Commission it is stated, on the authority of Dr. Frankland, that under the influence of this material (spongy iron) Thames water assumes the chemical characters of deep well water. It has been tried on a large scale at Antwerp, and proved to be remarkably efficient.

The Chamberland-Pasteur filter, recently introduced, would seem to be the best of all domestic filters. In its simplest form it consists of a tube of fine unglazed biscuit porcelain, which may be screwed on to the service tap, when the pressure of the water will force the fluid through the pores of the porcelain, and a fairly rapid rate of filtration results. It effectually strains off all organisms and their spores, but it has little or no effect on the chemical constituents in solution; its action is purely mechanical. The surface of the porcelain tube in a short time becomes covered with a slimy coating, even when an apparently clean water is filtered. This coating is, however, readily and quickly removed by taking out the tube and brushing it freely, or by washing it with dilute hydrochloric acid.

Reference must be made to a paper recently (January 18th, 1897) read by Mr. W. J. Dibdin on "The Character of the London Water Supply." He submitted tables showing the great bacteriological improvement which has taken place in the quality of the water between the years 1892 and 1895. The change had been so great that even the bacteria in the river itself at Sunbury had been reduced to one-tenth of their former number. The amount of sewage passing into the river above the Companies' intake must therefore have been greatly lessened. Mr. Dibdin had also investigated the effects of a well-known softening process upon the dissolved and undissolved impurities contained in Thames water. The process (known as Clark's) consists in the addition of lime, which, by combining with the carbonic acid, causes all the carbonate of lime previously held in solution to be thrown down. At the same time, the organic carbon and nitrogen are considerably reduced in quantity, and 87 per cent. of the bacteria are removed from the water, which, according to Mr. Dibdin, in respect of its chemical quality and number of bacteria, is thereby improved to a degree comparable with that of the Welsh sources.

If we leave the theories of chemists and turn to matters of fact, we find that the inhabitants of the metropolis have been drinking Thames water for many years, and that London is the healthiest large city in the civilised world. The germs of disease must have found their way over and over again into the water, and in such quantities as to have produced serious outbreaks, had they not been rendered harmless or destroyed. Attempts to connect excessive rates of mortality with impurity of Thames water have altogether failed; in fact, when the latter condition has existed, it has been noticed that the health of London was excellent, and the deaths far below the average.

If all the circumstances be dispassionately considered, there would appear to be no sufficient reason for rejecting the present sources of water supply and for seeking others. It is not, however, intended to imply that no improvements are necessary. The further development of the constant system of supply (so as to do away with cisterns) cannot be too strongly recommended; and the same may be said of a vigorous enforcement of the provisions of the "Rivers Pollution Act." Those who condemn Thames water have no doubt done good service, inasmuch as they have stimulated the companies to do their best with the present sources of supply. It is not of course denied that better water could be got from the lake districts of Wales and Cumberland, but the necessity for bringing water from such distances has never been demonstrated. There is one obvious way by which great improvements could be effected, and that is the transference of the metropolitan waterworks to a public authority. It is unfortunate that this plan, which was brought forward some years ago by Lord Cross, has not been carried into effect. The consolidation of establishments, the increased vigilance in collecting rates, with the consequent cheapness of the water, and the unity of action in effecting all necessary improvements, are a few of the advantages which would accrue from such a change. It is not too much to hope that some similar measure may ere long engage the earnest consideration of Parliament.

XII.

HEALTH-RESORTS AND THEIR USES.

THE idea that a remedy exists for every disease to which human beings are subject is one which must always be fascinating. We naturally regard diseases as so many enemies, and would fain persuade ourselves that Providence has placed within our reach certain agencies by which they may be subdued. At the same time one is forced to confess that every-day experience does not encourage these sanguine views. We look around us and see cases of chronic disease, little if at all benefited by the treatment of the most scientific character, carried out in the best possible manner. Still, with some, the idea survives that a remedy might be found if only we knew where to look for it. This notion was doubtless largely fostered by the implicit faith in drugs which prevailed not many decades ago, and is yet far from extinct. Such subjects as fresh pure air, diet, clothing, exercise, etc., now justly considered as of great moment, were for the most part either totally neglected or passed over as quite subordinate in value. The science of hygiene —that is, of the art of preserving health—has advanced with rapid strides since the beginning of this century, and more particularly during the last thirty years. While the treatment of disease by drugs has lost much of its popularity, an ever-increasing reliance is placed on hygienic measures and dietetic regulations. The first rank among the former must be accorded to what is termed " change of air," and to the various beneficial influences connected with that large class of localities known as " health-resorts." Such indeed is the estimate in the public mind of the value of health-resorts, and so boundless the promises made on behalf of so many of these places, that it would seem as though the idea not of one, but of a score of unfailing remedies for every disease, had been triumphantly realised. I propose to discuss, firstly, the principal uses of health-resorts and the expectations which may be formed in regard to them; and, secondly, to compare foreign health-resorts with those which are to be found in the British Islands.

The belief has prevailed from very early times that health could be restored by a sojourn in certain localities. It is probable that, as at the present day, a change of temperature constituted in most cases the principal attraction. The dwellers in a hot, enervating climate would find that improved health and vigour attended even a short visit to a region possessing climatic conditions of an opposite character; and on the other hand, sufferers from various disorders—*e.g.*, of the rheumatic class—found relief in the heat from which the former had been glad to escape. But besides differences of temperature, several circumstances, peculiar to a locality, exercise a special influence upon health. The pureness and freshness of the air, the existence of springs, the nature of the vegetation and of the soil, and the proximity to the sea, would be the chief points. A place marked out from the surrounding neighbourhood by the possession of any of these advantages, would in the course of time be regarded as a sanatorium, at all events for certain classes of diseases. The benefits which so often result from change of air, popularly so-called, are matters of daily experience, and are never more clearly exhibited than in cases of convalescence from acute and severe disorders. Unmistakable signs of improvement seldom fail to make their appearance, in a very short time, when convalescents—for instance, from fevers—are removed from the scenes of their illnesses into country air or to the seaside, which may be cited as instances in point. Various chronic conditions of ill-health are scarcely, if at all, relieved by medicine alone, whereas a change of air frequently brings about an improvement. In a large number of cases, the physical qualities of the atmosphere of certain districts and localities have a peculiarly beneficial and curative action, but different conditions are required by different persons. Just as the jaded dwellers in crowded cities are benefited by country air, so, as has been said, it is found that a temporary change of an opposite character, and apparently for the worse as regards hygienic surroundings, often produces similar results. When the mind is active and the disposition social, the tranquillity of a country life sometimes acts prejudicially upon the nervous system, and causes deterioration of health and strength. Under such circumstances restoration is best effected by removal to a town, where the mental faculties can find appropriate opportunities for exercise. The benefit in these cases is due really to the change of environment, and not to the hygienic qualities of the place. The same with regard to food. Persons to whom delicate and highly nutritious viands appear from long use to be absolutely necessary, frequently discover that coarser fare can be taken with relish, and that the digestion is thereby improved.

That the benefits often result from the change, and not necessarily from the place, is proved by the fact that a permanent residence in the locality does not always perpetuate the advantage gained during the earlier period of the sojourn. It is clear, therefore, that change of air includes many aids to health besides the physical properties of the atmosphere. In cases of convalescence from acute disease, it is true that much of the benefit derivable from change of air is due to minute differences in the physical constitution of the atmosphere. Modern chemical researches have shown that the air of cities and towns and the air of country places differ as regards the proportions of oxygen and carbonic acid. But generally, new scenes, agreeable society, recreation, rest, or at least freedom from toil and ordinary avocations, assist very considerably in the restoration of shattered nerves and broken health.

To estimate the popular opinion of the value of change of air, it is only necessary to cast a glance at the number of books written for the purpose of instructing the sick and their advisers in the choice of a locality, or of proclaiming the special advantages of particular places as regards climate, mineral springs, or other features. No department of hygiene has been so copiously treated as this. Caution is, however, necessary in accepting statements with reference to localities in which the authors have more or less interest. Great kindness is usually displayed towards the virtues of the place so confidently recommended, while its faults are conveniently kept in the background, or not allowed to exist. One of the handiest and most trustworthy works is Dr. Macpherson's "Baths and Wells of Europe." With this work and "Our Baths and Wells," by the same author, it is not difficult to form a practical judgment as to the real character of any given health-resort. Having come to the conclusion that a change of air is desirable or necessary, the important question to decide is, What locality offers the best chances of recovery or of prolongation of life? Various circumstances require consideration; the chief of these are, the ailment of the patient, his own desires, his pecuniary means, and his ability or otherwise to stand the fatigue of a journey. In some cases mere change of abode is sufficient; in others, a change from one part of England to another, as to the seaside, appears to fulfil all requirements; while, in a third class, certain advantages are connected with foreign travel and residence. In addition to the good results arising from change of air, there are those which are obtainable from drinking or bathing in the waters of certain localities, such waters either possessing a high temperature or containing an unusual proportion of certain saline matters in a state of solution, or exhibiting both these peculiarities.

It is not easy to give in a few words a proper definition of climate. The most obvious circumstances which affect the climate of a region or country are temperature, humidity, purity of the atmosphere, wind, atmospheric pressure, intensity of light, soil, amount of vegetation, and nearness to the sea. Many conditions, however, operate on the human system besides those which come under the cognisance of the meteorologist. Pure air, abundance of sunshine without excessive heat, so that several hours can be spent in the open air; an equable temperature and absence of, or shelter from, high winds, whether hot or cold, are the main *desiderata* for all classes of patients. For our present purpose, the most convenient division of climate is into that of (1) the seashore, (2) the mountains, (3) inland wooded districts, and (4) the open sea. The climate of the seashore presents several marked peculiarities. Owing to the continuous evaporation going on from the sea, the temperature during the summer months is lower than that of the neighbouring inland districts; it is also much more equable, because the sea water maintains its temperature for some time, in spite of changes of wind and other disturbing causes. The air from the sea also contains abundant moisture and particles of saline matter in suspension; it is more dense, and therefore a given volume contains more oxygen than ordinary air. Sea air also contains much ozone and a minute quantity of iodine. The effects of sea air are well known. It improves the digestive powers and promotes changes of the bodily tissues. It strengthens the nervous system, and hence it materially assists in the recovery from various forms of illness. These effects are for the most part rapidly produced.

Sea air is useful in almost all cases of chronic disease, and especially in those of tedious convalescence. When, however, the digestive and assimilative functions are very weak, the result is often not satisfactory, inasmuch as waste of the body is promoted, while a corresponding amount of new material fails to be assimilated. Under such circumstances a preliminary sojourn for a short period in pure country air is advisable. No country in the world can vie with England in the number and variety of its seaside places, many of them excellently situated, and offering every advantage in the way of fresh air, facilities for bathing, etc. These advantages are, however, much neglected, and sometimes turned into positive sources of mischief. It is a serious error to suppose that bathing in sea water is *always* innocuous and generally beneficial, and that in these respects it has the advantage over bathing in fresh water. Bathing in the open air is potent either for good or evil according to circumstances, yet it too often happens that baths are taken even by delicate persons without proper advice. As Dr. Weber points out, even warm sea-baths are generally indulged in more on the prompting of the inclination than under competent advice. He adds that, " infinite advantages might be derived from them, either alone or combined with the internal use of waters. Many invalids would gain more from such a plan properly carried out than from a visit to a continental spa." It certainly seems strange that whereas advice is always sought before taking baths at continental bathing-places, where perhaps the water contains only a small proportion of saline matter and differs but little from that of an ordinary warm bath, courses of warm sea-water baths in England are often taken by invalids of all kinds without any advice, and with blind confidence in the suitableness of the water to all conditions. Sea air is especially beneficial in scrofula, in bronchitis, in many cases of rheumatism, in gout, and in most cases of consumption. The increased temperature plays an important part in the alleviation of many of these diseases. The list of English summer health-resorts by the seaside is a very long one. Those on the eastern coast, from Tynemouth to Dover, have a comparatively dry and bracing climate. On the south-east, as far as the Isle of Wight, there are a host of well-known places with climates differing according to their situation, aspect, exposure to certain winds, etc. Further westward are

Bournemouth, so justly renowned as a winter-residence, Torquay, Penzance, etc. On the west coast are the Welsh watering-places, and those of Lancashire, Westmoreland, and Cumberland. Many very desirable spots are to be found on the coasts of Scotland—North Berwick, Dunoon, Nairn, Rothesay, and Ardrossan being those that are best known. Ireland is almost equally well provided with similar places. The Channel Islands have many qualities to recommend them, especially during the winter season. Their temperature is considerably higher and more equable than that of most portions of our southern coasts.

The diseases for which seaside stations are generally resorted to are pulmonary complaints, including consumption, bronchitis, and asthma. England is not deficient in localities eminently suitable for persons suffering from these affections. These localities are all characterised by mildness and equability of temperature, and purity and comparative calmness of the atmosphere. In the advantages they offer to patients suffering from pulmonary diseases they are second to few, and they have the marked recommendation of being easily accessible, near home, and within reach of friends. Of course as regards temperature they cannot compete with the Riviera, but temperature is not everything, even in the treatment of a consumptive patient. Indeed, from recent experience, it would seem that hot climates are not necessarily good for consumption, and that cold and frost are by no means always bad, but sometimes salutary for chest diseases. Moreover, we are assured by Dr. Bennet that the descriptions of the winter climate of Nice, Cannes, and Hyères, and of Italy in general, as contained in most books of travel, works on climate, and guide-books, are mere poetical delusions. "The perpetual spring, the eternal summer, the warm south, the balmy atmosphere," described in such glowing terms, exist only in the imagination of the writers.

Some of our English health-resorts have other recommendations beyond their temperature as curative agencies for chest diseases. Bournemouth, for example, combines several favourable conditions, met with elsewhere only at Arcachon. The natural purity of the air is secured at Bournemouth by the general adoption of stipulations for a large space round every house. The atmosphere of the place is positively disinfected by the "oxidising and antiseptic influences of the peroxide of hydrogen and camphoraceous matters, due to the chemical effect of moisture and sunshine upon the terebinthinate emanations from the pine-trees." Dr. Dobell has given figures showing that upwards of three million pine-trees remain in the different districts of Bournemouth and its immediate surroundings. These trees give off an immense quantity of camphoraceous material, the antiseptic powers of which car be conceived, if we reflect that a comparatively weak solution " is sufficiently strong to preserve animal matter almost indefinitely free from decomposition." The atmosphere is soothing to the respiratory organs, is mild and fairly equable, and not relaxing by over moisture. The night-temperature during winter is never very low ; fogs are unknown ; and, according to Dr. Dobell, the hotels, boarding-houses, and lodging-houses are, almost without exception, excellently built and well-arranged for invalids. When such advantages as these can be obtained near home, it is surely a mistake to send patients several hundred miles for the sake of a somewhat higher temperature. No doubt, to bask in the sunshine of the Riviera for several hours a day is most enjoyable and exhilarating; but at sunset the temperature rapidly falls, and a frosty night often succeeds a day on which the majority of invalids required sunshades to protect them from the heat. Unless proper care be taken, such variations of temperature are apt to lead to very untoward accidents.

Space will not permit me to dwell at greater length upon this topic, and I now pass on to consider another class of climates available as health-resorts, namely, that of mountains. The term "mountain-climate" is generally applicable in Europe to heights of from 1,500 to 6,000 feet. The effect of mountain air resembles in some respects that of sea air. The differences are for the most part due to lower density and temperature, and to the more frequent variations in the latter respect. The air also contains less moisture, and the temperature often falls considerably at night. The effect of mountain air is to improve the digestion and nutrition, and to strengthen the nervous system. The improvement in these respects is brought about less rapidly than at the seaside. Owing to the rarefaction of the air with the increase of elevation, more frequent and deeper inspirations are required, and more or less excitement of the organs of circulation necessarily ensues. Mountain climates are suitable for many cases of convalescence from acute diseases, and for conditions of ill-health in which want of tone is the prevailing characteristic. Where there is great muscular debility, or any organic disease of the heart, such climates are decidedly unsuitable. Of late years several mountainous localities have obtained a considerable reputation for the treatment of cases of consumption, and of these Davos Platz is perhaps the most celebrated. This place is 4,800 feet above the sea-level, and six or seven hours by *diligence* from Landquart Station, on the road from Zurich to Coire. Its efficacy for the cure of consumption in the case of natives of the lowland stations has long been known. Evidence of the value of mountain air in consumption has also been derived from the experience of medical practitioners in the large towns at the base of the Peruvian Andes. Consumption appears to be a very common disease in these places, and the removal of the patients to stations at elevations of several thousand feet is attended by the happiest results. The winter climate at Davos is preferable to that of the summer, as there is far less wind, and the climate is more equable and dry. Snow begins to fall in November, and continues through December, generally attaining a depth of three or four feet. "The atmosphere," says Dr. Burney Yeo, "becomes still and calm, the air intensely cold and dry, and absolutely clear. The temperature at night often falls very low, frequently some degrees below zero. The days are cloudless, with an intensely blue sky, and an amount of heat from solar radiation which enables invalids to pass hours sitting in the open air; and the brilliancy of the sunshine in midwinter makes umbrellas and sunshades essential for protection."

South Africa possesses many stations the natural conditions of which render them very suitable for the treatment of affections of the chest. One region, called the Karroo (signifying the dryness of the climate), is pre-eminent in this respect. It is divided into two portions, termed the Great and the Northern Karroo. The former consists of a vast plateau of considerable elevation, averaging about 3,000 feet above the level of the sea, whilst the average height of the mountain ranges is about 5,000 feet, some places rising to 7,000. Its special character is its excessive dryness—it is said that a clean polished steel razor can be left out all night in the open without fear of its acquiring one single speck of rust. Rain falls very irregularly, and at rare intervals only, and in small local showers—many months may elapse without a drop of rain. The atmosphere is pure and wonderfully exhilarating. The summer temperature, though high, is easily tolerated; the winter is cold, but bright and bracing, with abundant sunshine. Among the places best adapted for sanatoria are Ceres (1,493 feet), Matjesfontein, Beaufort West, and Cradock, all at an elevation of nearly 3,000 feet. The Northern Karroo lies at a much greater elevation than the Great Karroo, averaging about 4,000 feet above the sea-level, while some of the mountain ranges reach 7,800 feet. Its atmosphere is characterised by peculiar dryness, which, in conjunction with the rarefaction, the constant sunlight, and its generally uniform character, endows the climate with properties obtainable in Europe only at much higher altitudes. Chest affections are rare, and consumption is almost unknown among the inhabitants born and bred in this region. The district can boast of a long list of stations, all of which may be strongly recommended as regards climate and natural advantages. Among them may be mentioned Frazerberg (4,500), Richmond, Victoria (West), Hanover, Aliwal (North), and Kimberley, all at an elevation of from 4,000 to 4,500 feet.

All these places—and many others might be added—possess a climate which experience has proved to be highly curative to consumptive patients. It is likewise beneficial in cases of debility and want of tone, many examples of which are to be found in our own country, especially that form of general tiredness with insomnia resulting from the wear and tear of modern life. But climate *per se* will not suffice; there are other factors which are equally necessary. It is within the knowledge of everybody that the diet of sufferers from consumption and other wasting disorders, should be as sustaining and nutritious as they can take or bear. In the cases referred to, the appetite is often capricious, and the amount of food taken is altogether insufficient to counterbalance the daily losses. Hence one important aim in treatment is to improve the appetite and digestion, and this object may often be attained by a sojourn in pure mountain air. But it is useless and almost cruel to stimulate the appetite, unless proper means of satisfying it can at the same time be secured, and in many of the places mentioned above there is a great defect in this respect, as well as in other matters of hygiene. In some letters which appeared in the *Standard* newspaper (1895), it was pointed out that in the "parts of South Africa suitable, as regards climate, for consumptive patients, comfortable quarters, good, wholesome, well-cooked food, and kindly attention are an unknown combination. Up-country hotels, even those advertising for invalids, are primarily bars and canteens, ill-adapted for delicate people. Small 'Sanatoria' have been started, but none have yet arisen in which the invalid is the first consideration, or with sufficient capital to place comfort and good food within reach of the invalid."

It is pleasant to be able to state that this drawback will soon cease to exist. While in South Africa, during the autumn of 1895, I had opportunities of discussing the subject with Mr. Cecil Rhodes, and later on, by his desire, with Mr. Lawrence, of Kimberley; and since my return Mr. Lawrence has forwarded to me, by Mr. Rhodes' request, gratifying reports embodying the ideas which were discussed at our interviews. The resolution, emanating from Mr. Rhodes, was speedily adopted, of establishing a sanatorium at Kimberley for the treatment of persons suffering from pulmonary complaints, especially in the incipient stages. Mr. Rhodes promised a contribution of £4,000 from some funds at his disposal, and £1,000 from his own purse. Another letter informs me that Mr. Rhodes has promised an additional £5,000. Such public-spirited generosity is deserving of the highest praise; the money could not be devoted to a better purpose.

Small institutions for the reception of invalids already exist, but in few, if any, are the arrangements of an altogether satisfactory character. A model sanatorium of the kind now proposed will not only be a source of benefit to those who can avail themselves of it, but will stimulate the foundation of similar institutions in suitable localities, and will indicate to all concerned the necessary conditions for the attainment of favourable results. Kimberley, the station chosen for the erection of the buildings, presents many advantages. Its climate is equal to that of any health-resort in South Africa, and its surroundings are generally better than can be found elsewhere. Among its advantages may be enumerated various clubs, the library, the theatre, and other places of amusement; also opportunities for golf, tennis, cricket, coursing and shooting, and the proximity of the river. The nuisance due to the dust (of which I can speak by personal experience), at Johannesburg and other localities, has been greatly lessened at Kimberley since the present water supply was obtained. The management of the Kimberley Sanatorium will be vested in a Board, several members of which, well-known Kimberley men, occupying the highest public and social positions in the town, have been already nominated. There will be a medical representative at Cape Town from whom patients arriving from Europe will be able to obtain all requisite information and advice. The fees for admission will be such as to secure a fair remuneration to the resident custodians. Large profits will not be aimed at, but the tariff will probably be a little higher than at ordinary hotels—with which the institution will compare favourably as regards comforts and necessaries for invalids. Admission will be granted only to those patients whose condition promises a fair chance of recovery. A sum of £8,000 has been set aside for the building, and plans have been invited by advertisement. I cannot but express my sincere gratification at having been associated in any degree with the inception of so benevolent and desirable a project.

It must appear strange, and to some extent inexplicable, that consumption should be cured, or at all events its symptoms brought to a standstill, and the general health vastly improved, by such different climates as those of

Davos, the Karroo, Torquay, Bournemouth, Mentone, Madeira, and other places. There are, however, several circumstances which serve as a tolerably adequate explanation, though it must be confessed that our predictions of the benefits likely to be derived in a given case from any particular locality are often falsified by the results. But the localities just mentioned have several features in common. The air is pure and free from admixture of organic particles. There is at these places an unusual amount of sunshine, so that patients can often spend several hours of each day in the open air, whereby the lungs are improved, the appetite and powers of digestion are increased, and the nervous system is strengthened. As to the special curative agencies at work in mountainous health-resorts, in addition to the dryness, purity, and stillness of the air, the freedom from organic particles, which we now know are active promoters of putrefaction, is in all probability the condition most potent for good in chest cases. There is also the rarefaction of the air, which causes more frequent and deeper inspirations, and thus improves the condition of the breathing apparatus. The healthy portions of the lung are called upon to display increased activity, and their action compensates for the loss of those portions invaded by disease. Besides these advantages, patients take more care of themselves in these elevated health-resorts than at others where the conditions more resemble those of ordinary life; the place and its peculiarities constitute a very important part of the treatment, and the regulations with regard to exposure, etc., are certain to be carefully attended to. It is only necessary to add that consumption is a disease of which there are several varieties, each having certain stages, and that the choice of the most suitable locality can be arrived at only after a thorough consideration of all the circumstances of the case.

A few words will suffice for the description of the climates of inland wooded districts and of the benefits to be derived therefrom. All large cities and towns are surrounded by more or less salubrious country places, a sojourn in which often serves to restore or improve the health. The pureness of the atmosphere and the comparative absence of organic particles are the principal favourable agencies at work. The air, too, is somewhat warmer and more equable; the humidity in wooded districts is higher. Such conditions are especially suited for convalescents from acute diseases, and for the improvement of chronic ailments. A change into country air, as has been hinted, may often be advantageously adopted as a preliminary to a lengthened sojourn by the seaside or a journey to a mountainous healthresort. But country air has a value of its own. Dr. Beale says, " If patients could be induced to retire to a pleasant part of the country, where they would take moderate exercise, and be free from mental anxiety, meet with agreeable society, live regularly, take small doses of alkalies, and bathe themselves for an hour or two a day in warm water, in which some carbonate of soda has been dissolved, they would receive as great a benefit as by travelling hundreds of miles away, and at much less trouble and expense." All this is no doubt true, but, as a general rule, persons like to find things ready to their hand, and put less trust in arrangements which could be made almost anywhere than in those which are the special characteristics of certain places. There are many localities to be found in England, Wales, and Scotland, specially adapted for all the purposes of summer health-resorts; but generally there are no proper hotels or establishments for the reception of numerous visitors; and such establishments are mostly discouraged by the landed proprietors, who occupy the most eligible localities. "Such," Dr. Weber points out, "is the case with the moors of Scotland and Yorkshire, with their wonderfully enlivening air. A small inn, a few cottages and scattered houses, rarely disengaged, are all that is to be had; and the social element is wanting, even if one be fortunate enough to obtain accommodation." Many localities close to London would afford most excellent summer health-resorts; in Surrey, for instance, the hills near Leith Hill, and the Ewhurst Windmill and Ranmore Common, near Dorking, or the Hindhead or the Blackdown, near Haslemere; while further away there are the South Downs, Dartmoor, and Cannock Chase. Little or no accommodation is, however, to be met with at any of these places.

The last form of climate to which allusion has been made is that of the open sea. Long sea voyages are of great value in many cases of consumption. The patients have the advantages of the constant influences of the sea air, combined with mental repose and passive exercise. There are, of course, several drawbacks, the most prominent being the liability to sea-sickness and to bad weather and the confinement which necessarily occurs; the monotony in occupations, the want of variety of food and of articles sometimes longed for by invalids, and the discomforts arising from the machinery, in the case of steam-vessels. If the patient be not liable to suffer from sea-sickness, and if his appetite and digestion be fair, he has a much better chance of being benefited by a sea voyage than under opposite conditions. Various conditions of debility, especially those arising from excessive mental strain, are almost certain to be improved by a sea voyage.

An important class of health-resorts includes those which have obtained their renown by reason of the possession of springs of water, valuable either on account of their temperature or because they contain an unusual amount of certain gaseous or saline matters in a state of solution. An enormous number of springs are now in vogue, and if we could believe a tithe of the statements confidently put forth as to their efficacy, chronic disease would be the fate only of those who either could not or would not visit the health-giving springs. Making allowances for an enormous amount of exaggeration, let us see what can be claimed for baths and waters. There is, however, a difficulty at the outset, inasmuch as it is impossible to separate the influence of such agencies as travelling, change of air, diet, and social conditions, from that which may be due to the external and internal use of any given water.

It is not easy to classify mineral waters, but for practical purposes they may be divided into seven groups. The first includes the *thermal* waters, which are characterised by considerable elevation of temperature and poorness in saline constituents; heat and purity are, in fact, their main peculiarities. By way of comparison, it may be desirable to mention that water artificially heated to from $85°$ to $92°$ constitutes a *tepid* bath; a *warm* bath has a temperature of from 92° to 98°; and a *hot* bath of from 98° to 104°. The best known thermal springs are those of Bath, Buxton, Teplitz, Gastein, Leuk, and Wildbad; the highest temperature of any of them being about 120°. When these slightly mineralised thermal waters are taken internally, the effect is neither more nor less than that of an equal quantity of ordinary water heated to the same temperature: tissue-change is promoted, and the action of those organs which remove waste products from the blood is increased. Hot water taken slowly is rapidly absorbed, and is useful for the purposes just mentioned. It is, however, in the form of baths that the simple thermal waters are mostly used, the effects depending on the temperature of the water and the time spent in the bath. The beneficial results of a course of warm baths are well known; the skin is softened and purified, more blood circulates in it, and its functions are promoted; the nervous system is soothed, and certain forms of swelling and exudation are lessened or removed. All these good effects are often witnessed in cases of rheumatism, gout, neuralgia, and likewise after injuries, especially of joints. It must be kept in mind that the warmth and the moisture are the curative agencies. In this class of waters there is no claim that any saline matters are absorbed by the skin; indeed, the quantity dissolved is too small to produce any effect, even were we to admit the possibility of absorption.

In connection with baths of all kinds, the capacity of the skin to absorb saline or other substances dissolved in the water is a point of considerable importance. All the tissues of the body are more or less porous, and therefore capable of soaking up water and various other fluids brought into contact with them. There is, it would appear, slight increase of weight after a *protracted* warm bath, and this is due to the imbibition of a certain quantity of water. As a matter of fact, however, the absorptive power of the skin is not great, and for this reason the integument constitutes a very effective barrier to the admission of materials into the blood. So long as the epidermis is intact, the hands can be dipped into solutions of poisonous substances without any risks of those evil results which would certainly follow the introduction of a similar fluid into the stomach. If it be true that only water is absorbed by the skin, the utility of bathing in iron waters or in alkaline waters, with the view of obtaining any *special benefit* from the *substances held in solution*, is clearly very questionable. Many experiments have been made for the purpose of determining this question. Highly soluble substances, such as iodide of potassium, have been added to baths of warm water and, after *prolonged immersion*, no trace of the iodine could be detected in the saliva. When, on the other hand, a few grains of this drug are dissolved in water and swallowed, the iodine can soon be discovered in the saliva by a simple test. It is true that certain medicines readily pass into the system when rubbed into the skin, but this method of application is different from simply keeping the skin in contact with substances dissolved in water. Curious properties have been assigned to thermal springs, owing, as has been thought, to some peculiarity of the heat. There is, however, no foundation for this view; water artificially heated to a given temperature is just as efficacious as that derived from springs destitute of any special character. This fact is sometimes disputed by those whose interest it is to advocate the claims of certain springs, but those who know most about such matters have little doubt as to its truth. Some years ago the local authorities at Wildbad (one of the best-known baths of this kind) were proposing to enlarge the bathing accommodation. One member of the Board objected to the proposal, alleging that any one could have a Wildbad bath in his back kitchen. We have in England one of the finest thermal springs to be found in Europe. For all cases for which hot baths are suggested, the waters of Bath are not to be surpassed, while all the arrangements for bathing fulfil every possible requirement. They are now regaining their reputation, having been undeservedly eclipsed by such places as Teplitz, Gastein, and Wildbad.

The next important group of mineral waters includes those which contain iron. These are used both for drinking and bathing purposes, but, as already mentioned, when taken as baths, they have no special virtues, inasmuch as the iron is not absorbed by the skin. For internal administration, however, they constitute most valuable remedies for all cases in which iron is indicated. In England we have but few springs of this character which are made any use of; that of Tunbridge Wells is probably the best known. It is used only for drinking purposes. One spring at Harrogate contains iron. At Llandrindod, in Radnorshire, there is a weak chalybeate spring, whose waters are said to be very decidedly tonic and hæmatinic, and easily assimilated. A few springs in various parts of England contain so much iron as to be unfit for internal use. On the Continent, the iron waters of Spa, Pyrmont, Schwalbach, and St. Moritz are those most resorted to. Many of these contain a large amount of free carbonic acid, and are on that account pleasant to take.

Sulphur waters form a third and distinct group, and we have in England, at Harrogate, one of the strongest of this class. In addition to sulphur, the waters of Harrogate contain a large amount of salts, the action of which cannot be separated from that of the sulphur.

Other sulphur springs are to be found at Strathpeffer and Llandrindod. On the Continent the springs at Aix-la-Chapelle and Aix-les-Bains are those that have the highest reputation. The sulphur waters are supposed to be useful in rheumatism, gout, neuralgia, liver disorders, various affections of the skin, and in sundry other diseases. Very divergent opinions are held as to their real value in any of these ailments. When taken as baths, their effects are probably identical with those of common water of an equal temperature, and the same, in my opinion, may be said with regard to their internal use. It is especially worthy of notice that those local physicians who are so enthusiastic over the virtues of these waters almost invariably order powerful medicines to be taken during the course of bathing and drinking. This custom is universal in their treatment of one class of patients who are sent in great numbers to Aix-la-Chapelle. Experience teaches us that the same medicines are wonderfully efficacious at home, without the addition of malodorous waters.

A fourth class of waters consists of those

which contain common salt as their principal constituent, and we have in England excellent representatives of this class. At Droitwich, Nantwich, and Middlewich, springs of brine are abundantly found, and the preparation of salt, by evaporating the liquor, forms the staple industry of these places. Brine from Droitwich has now been conveyed to Malvern, where patients have the advantages of using the strongest possible saline baths in a health-resort celebrated for its dry air, perfectly pure water, and exquisite scenery. The arrangements at Malvern are excellent, and well adapted for invalids. The water is too highly saline for internal use, but in the form of baths the salt acts as a powerful stimulant to the skin, and promotes its nutrition. By its action on the cutaneous nerves, it gives tone to the system. Springs of water containing much common salt are also to be found at Cheltenham, Leamington, and Llandrindod; at Kreuznach, Rehme, and many other places on the Continent. Alkaline waters, which owe their properties to the presence of carbonate of soda, are not to be found in England. The most celebrated are those of Vichy, Neuenahr, and

Mont Doré, which are hot, and those of Bilin, Apollinaris, Vals, and Taunus, which are cold. This class of waters enjoys a considerable reputation in the treatment of indigestion and of those conditions in which an undue amount of acid is present in the system—*e.g.*, in rheumatism and gout. They are used both for bathing and drinking, though, as stated in a previous paragraph, no appreciable amount of the saline matters is absorbed by the skin. Their internal use promotes tissue-change, and if continued for some time produces emaciation. It must be admitted that under their use the symptoms of chronic gout and rheumatism are often much relieved, but with regard especially to the former affection, these alkaline waters act merely as palliatives, the symptoms sooner or later recurring when their use is discontinued. On this account they are far inferior to such waters as those of Carlsbad, which belong to a class to be next described. When taken by gouty persons, the alkaline waters—*e.g.*, of Vichy—neutralise the *materies morbi*, but have little, if any, influence in checking its formation. The Carlsbad waters, on the other hand, while neutralising the offending material, act likewise upon those organs which are concerned in its production in such a manner that its formation is decidedly checked.

The next class of waters, those which contain the sulphates of soda and magnesia, is now represented in England chiefly by the springs of Cheltenham and Leamington, though there are many others which contain these salts. Springs at Epsom, Streatham, and Dulwich were very highly thought of in the last century. Nowadays we import large quantities of weaker waters, such as Püllna, Friedrichshall, Hunyadi Yanos, etc. These are highly useful in many cases. The Carlsbad waters, already referred to, contain, beside sulphates, the carbonate of soda, and are therefore more suitable for many cases than those just mentioned.

The last class of waters which require notice is not a numerous one. It contains those springs of which the chief mineral constituents are the carbonates and sulphates of lime and magnesia. We have no representative of this class in England; abroad, the best known springs are those of Bagnères de Bigorre,

Contrexéville, and Wildungen. They are useful in some forms of indigestion, especially where acidity is a prominent symptom, and in some skin diseases. As baths, their effects are due simply to the heat and the water. No absorption of the salts can be supposed to take place.

This necessarily imperfect sketch of health-resorts and their uses is sufficient to show that we have in such places remedial agencies of a very potent character. We must beware, however, of expecting impossibilities and of falling into the mistake of supposing that the majority of ailments are curable by baths and waters. It is unfortunately impossible to obtain any statistics as to the results in the thousands of patients who annually visit baths and watering-places, either by the advice of physicians or prompted by their own ideas of what will be good for them. Favourable cases are of course published in the local handbooks; we hear nothing of the majority who fail to obtain relief. With regard to baths, it would seem at least probable that foreigners in general are more often benefited than Englishmen, to whom daily ablution is not such a novelty as it must be as a general rule to dwellers on the Continent. A glance at the utensils provided for washing in most continental hotels is sufficient to show the slight attention ordinarily paid to this important part of the toilet. Judging from the writer's experience, it is necessary to add that all patients hoping to derive real benefit from a health-resort should seek proper advice before resorting thither, and that, while there, they should follow out to the letter the advice of the local physician. Unless his directions, trivial as they may seem, are attended to, the place and its resources will not have a fair trial. It must be borne in mind that in not a few cases the improvement shows itself only after the patient has returned home. There is nothing surprising in this delay, as most of the ailments, for the relief of which recourse is had to bathing-places, are of a chronic nature, and do not admit of rapid cure. Lastly, when a health-resort has to be selected, let it never be forgotten that our country possesses many places of this character, and in no respect second to those to be found abroad.

INDEX.

Abraham, age at his death, 62.
Abstainers, total, longevity of, 133; compared with moderate drinkers, 134; two classes of, 135.
Actuaries, Institute of, tables of longevity, 64.
Addison, Dr., on diphtheria, 165.
Addison, J., on the valetudinarian, 87.
Africa, production of intoxicating drinks, 114.
—— South, places suitable for affections of the chest, 326-328; defective arrangements for invalids, 329.
Air, conductivity of, 104; a purifier of water, 292; benefits from change of, 312-315; sea, 318; bathing, 319; mountain, 324; country, 334; sea voyages, 337.
Aix-la-Chapelle, 344.
Aix-les-Bains, 344.
Alcohol, use of, 49, 85, 113; manufacture, 114; general action, 115; excitement, 115-117; intoxication, 117; coma or insensibility, 118; effects on the body, 119; on the nervous system, 119; sedative effects, 121; wine, spirits, and beer compared, 123; absorption, 125; acts as a food, 126; compared with opium, 127; reasons for taking, 129; question of necessity, 130; rate of mortality, 133; abstinence contrasted with moderation, 133-136; quantity, 136; tendency to retard digestion, 139.
Aldershot, result of the antitoxin treatment at, 186.
Aliwal, 328.
Alkaline waters, 345.
America, extension of diphtheria to, 168.
American children, causes of ill-health, 39.
Andes, Peruvian, 326.
Animals, fasting, experiments on, 146; diphtheria in, 179.

INDEX.

Anthrax or splenic fever, 235; experiments on the organisms, 236.
Antitoxin, value of, 7; discovery, 183; method of preparation, 183; results of the treatment, 185.
Apollinaris, 346.
Arcachon, 322.
Ardrossan, 321.
Aretæus, his description of diphtheria, 167.
Arnold, Matthew, on the use of alcohol, 122.
Artesian well, the first, 298.
Assurance offices, statistics on total abstinence, 133.
Australia, effects of the antitoxin treatment in, 185.
Austria, effect of the antitoxin treatment in, 185.

BACILLUS of cholera, 205, 207; size, 205; mode of transport, 208; growth and development, 209.
—— of diphtheria, 175.
Bacon, Lord, on the pleasures of gardening, 82.
Bacteria, nature and mode of growth, 205; formation of spores or seeds, 205; qualities, 206; forms of action, 207; theory of, 231; meaning of the term, 231; the common form, 232; existence of, in water, 301; test by cultivation, 302; development in filtered or unfiltered, 303; reduction of, 306.

Bagnères de Bigorre, 347.
Barnard Castle, 292.
Barrister, the daily work of a, 17-20.
Batavia, 201.
Bath, thermal springs at, 339, 342.
Bathing, 319.
Baths, results of warm, 339.
Battersea, mortality from cholera, 193, 195.
Beale, Dr., on particles of contagious bioplasm, 229, 230; on the value of country air, 335.
Beaufort West, 327.
Bedroom, temperature of, 90.
Beer, amount of alcohol in, 124.
Behring, 184.
Bengal, epidemic of cholera, in 1817, 188.
Bennet, Dr., on the climate of Italy, 322.
Bermondsey, mortality from cholera, 194.
Bertillon, Dr., on marriage affecting longevity, 68.
Berwick, North, 321.
Bicycling, the exercise of, 82.
Bilin, 346.
Bioplasm, 229.
Birmingham, epidemic of diphtheria, 168.
Bischof, Prof., on water from wells, 297; the development of bacteria in water, 303.
Blackdown, 336.
Blackwall, 201.
Body, normal temperature, 95; variations, 95; preservation of

INDEX.

the general level, 96; loss of heat, 97; use of clothing, 98.
Boulogne sore throat, **epidemic of**, in 1855, 165, 169; number of deaths from, 166.
Bournemouth, 321, 333; advantages of, 322.
Brain, **weakness of**, 15.
Brandy, analysis of, 123.
Bretonneau, M., his use of the term diphtheria, 166, 169.
Brighton, 54.
Bristol, the sewers of, 172.
British Medical Association, report of the Investigation Committee, 85.
Bromine, 256.
Bromley, mortality from diphtheria, 168.
Brunton, Dr., on the effects of alcohol, 116, 117.
Bryson, Dr., on the outbreak of cholera on board ship, 200.
Budd, Dr. W., 300.
Buffon on the normal duration of human life, 61.
Bulwer on light reading, 52.
Burnett's solution of chloride of zinc, 260.
Buxton, thermal springs, 339.

CABINET Minister, the work of a, 25.
Cannes, 322.
Cannock Chase, 336.
Carbolic acid, 212, 257, 263.
Carlsbad waters, 346, 347.
Carpenter, Dr. W. B., 132, 142.
Caterham epidemic, 293, 300.

Cats, diphtheria in, 180.
Ceres, 327.
Chadwell, 277.
Chadwick, Sir Edwin, example of transmitted longevity, 67.
Chamberland-Pasteur filters, 214, 265, 305.
Champagne, its intoxicating power, 123.
Change of air, 311: *see* Air.
Channel Islands, 321.
Charcoal filters, 265.
Chelsea, mortality from cholera, 193.
Chelsea Water Company, 277.
Cheltenham, 345, 347.
Chesham, Bucks, epidemic of diphtheria, 168.
Chevreul, M., age at his death, 93: *note*.
Chinese method of clothing, 105.
Chingford, 277.
Chloride of zinc, 260, 263.
Chlorine gas, use of, 245, 254, 264.
Cholera, epidemics of, in India, 187-190; theories of its origin, 191; effect of impure water, 192; epidemics in London, 1849, 193; 1854, 194, 195; 1866, 195; theory of air-conduction, 199; outbreaks of, on board ship, 200-202; controversies on the subject, 203; invisible animalcules, 204; the bacilli, 204; special precautions, 210-214; general rules for the prevention of, 214; method of inoculating, 216.

23

Chossat, M., his experiments on fasting animals, 146, 149.
Cleanliness, importance of, 90.
Clergy, average duration of life, 68.
Clergy Mutual Assurance, 135.
Climate, definition of, 317.
Clothing, use of, 98; wool, 98; shoddy, 99; silk, 101; fur, 101; felt, 101; cotton, 102; linen, 102; the best material, 102; colour, 108; waterproof, 108; general rules for, 110.
Coffee, the use of, 130.
Coire, 325.
Combermere, Lord, 73.
Companies, water, 277: *see* Water.
Competition, the strain of, 28.
Condy's fluid, 259.
Consumption, localities suitable for, 321, 322, 325, 328, 332.
Contagion synonymous with infection, 219.
Contrexéville, 348.
Cornwall, epidemic of diphtheria, 168.
Corrosive sublimate, 211, 257.
Cotton, an important article of clothing, 102; its conducting power, 103.
Country air, value of, 334.
Cows, diphtheria in, 179.
Cradock, 327.
Crayford, 277.
Crookshank, Dr., 258.
Cross, Lord, 309.

DALGETTY, CAPTAIN, 45.

Darlington, 292.
Dartmoor, 336.
Davaine, his experiments on anthrax, 235.
Davos Platz, its efficacy for the cure of consumption, 325, 333; climate, 326.
De Quincey on the different effects of opium and alcohol, 127.
Delirium tremens, 120.
Delta, outbreaks of cholera, 187.
Deodorisation, 245.
Deptford, 277.
Descartes, his plan of prolonging life, 73.
Desmond, Lady, her reputed longevity, 63.
Devonshire, epidemic of diphtheria, 168.
Dibdin, Mr. W. J., his paper on "The Character of the London Water Supply," 306.
Diet suitable for aged persons, 84.
Digby, Sir Kenelm, 73.
Digestion, state of the, 45; process, 46; diet, 49; effects of alcohol, 138.
Dinner hour, 47.
Diphtheria, outbreak of, in 1856, 164; derivation of the word, 166; prevalence in early times, 167; in Spain, 167; in England, 168; characteristics, 169; average mortality, 170; sanitary measures, 171; variety of causes for the development,

INDEX. 355

172-174; liability of children, 174; the bacillus, 175; contagious character, 175; propagation by elementary schools, 176; milk, 178; animals, 179; notification, 180; isolation, 181; treatment, 182; discovery of antitoxin, 183; result of the treatment, 185.

Disinfection, meaning of the word, 218; ancient method, 243; adoption of deodorants, 245; modern rules, 247, 261-265; high temperature, 248; difficulties of the process, 249-251; exposure to light and air, 251; washing, 252, 263; rooms, 253; various methods, 253-260, 264; ventilation, 253; chlorine, 254; euchlorine, 255; bromine, 256; bread, 256; spray, 257; carbolic acid, 257; Condy's fluid, 259; sinks, drains, etc., 260.

Distilled water, 285.
Ditton, 277.
Dobell, Dr., on the advantages of Bournemouth, 323.
Doré, Mont, 346.
Dorunda, outbreak of cholera on board, 200.
Dover, 320.
Drains, disinfection of, 260.
Droitwich, 345.
Drugs, injurious use of, 30; faith in, 311.
Dulwich, 347.
Dunoon, 321.
Dynamometer, 161.

EARLY rising, the practice of, 43-45.
Eastbourne, 54.
Easton, extract from his work on " Human Longevity," 61.
England, number of deaths from diphtheria, 170.
England, outbreak of cholera on board, 202.
Epsom, 347.
Esmarch, Prof., on the use of bread in disinfection, 256.
Euchlorine, 255, 262.
Ewhurst windmill, 336.
Exercise of the mind, 77; of the body, 79; need for discretion, 80; various forms of, 81.

FAKIRS, cases of suspended animation, 156.
Fasting, 144; symptoms of, in animals, 146; loss of weight, 147; cause of death, 148; cases of voluntary abstinence, 149-155; suspended animation, 155; symptoms of, in human beings, 156-158; loss of weight, 159; fall of temperature, 160.
Felt, 101.
Fevers, example of infectious, 220; of non-infectious, 222.
Filters, 213, 265, 304.
Fire, its use in disinfection, 243.
Fish, increase in the use of, 49.
Foderé, his case of starvation, 154.
Food, improvement in the method of preparing, 49; moderation in, 83; two classes of, 112.

Fothergill, Dr. J., 168.
France, effects of the antitoxin treatment in, 185.
Frankland, Dr. Percy, his report on the quality of water, 282, 283, 284, 302; on oxidation, 291; report on Tees river, 292; on two systems of water supply, 294; average reduction of organisms, 304.
Frazerberg, 328.
Fresh air, importance of 50.
Friedrichshall, 347.
Fungi, 230.
Fur, use of, 101.

GARDENING, a form of exercise, 82.
Garottillo, 167.
Gastein, thermal springs, 339, 342.
Germany, effects of the antitoxin treatment in, 185.
Gladstone, Mr., 33.
Golden Square, Soho, outbreak of cholera, in 1854, 195.
Grand Junction Water Company, 277.
Grand, Mr. A. le, on the purification of water exposed to air, 292.
Greeks, duration of life in the time of, 63.
Greenwich, mortality from diphtheria, 168.
Greg, Mr., 13; on a life without leisure, 32.

HAFFKINE, M., his method of anti-cholera vaccination, 216.

Halifax, 202.
Hamburg, epidemic of cholera, 209.
Hammersmith, mortality from cholera, 193.
Hampton, 277.
Hanover, 328.
Hanwell Asylum well, 299.
Hardy, Sir J. Duffus, on the longevity of man in the Middle Ages, 63.
Harrogate, 343.
Health, undue solicitude for, 87.
Health resorts, value of, 311; benefits from change of air, 312-315; character of localities, 316; effects of sea-air, 318; bathing, 319; list of seaside places, 320; equability of temperature, in chest diseases, 321; advantages of Bournemouth, 322; mountain air, 324; Davos Platz, 325; South Africa, 326-328; Kimberley Sanatorium, 331; effect on consumption, 332; country air, 334; localities, 336; sea voyages, 337; mineral waters and baths, 338-348.
Heat, loss of, 97; conducting power of clothing materials, 103; of air, 104.
Hereditary longevity, 67.
High-pressure, evidences of, 27; symptoms, 29; results, 33.
Hindhead, 336.
Hirsch, Dr., on diphtheria, 174.
Hogarth on the difference

between topers and dram-drinkers, 125.

Holidays, 53; mode of spending the annual, 55.

Holland, Sir H., on the habit of early rising, 72.

Holmes, Wendell, on the use of alcohol, 122.

Hook, Dean, 44; on the practice of reading, 52.

Horses, use of, for the antitoxin serum, 183.

Howard, John, on the insanitary condition of prisons, 3.

Hufeland on longevity, 67.

Humphry, Sir G. M., his statistics on fifty-two centenarians, 64, 71; extract from his "Report on Aged Persons," 69, 83.

Hunyadi Yanos, 347.

Hurdwar, outbreaks of cholera, 187.

Hyères, 322.

Hygiene, personal, 8; advancement in the science of, 311.

"Hypochondriasis," 31, 87.

ICED water, injurious use of, 49.

India, epidemics of cholera, 187-189; use of water, 274.

Indian Archipelago, production of intoxicating drinks, 114.

Indigestion, 30; number of remedies for, 46.

Infection, meaning of the word, 218; typical example of, 220; of non-infection, 222; distinction as regards causation, 225; differences in the nature of contagious agencies, 227; nature of particles, 228; *bioplasm*, 229; *fungi*, 230; *bacteria*, 231; relation between the organisms and symptoms, 233; protective inoculation, 239; media for the propagation, 241; fatal character, 243.

Inoculation, protective, 7, 239.

Insanity, increase of, 31.

Intoxication, 117.

Iodide of potassium, 341.

Iron waters, 342.

Irwell river, 291.

JACKSON, DR. H., 32.

Jacobs, Sarah, her death from starvation, 151.

Jameson, Dr., 192.

Japanese method of clothing, 105.

Jenkins, Henry, his reputed longevity, 63.

Jenner, Edward, the first to practice vaccination in 1796, 5; his view of its protective powers, 6.

Johannesburg, 331.

Johnson, Dr., on the advantages of living in London, 11.

Joshua, age at his death, 62.

Judge, the duties of a, 20.

KARROO, the Great, 327; the Northern, 327.

Kent Waterworks Company, 277, 280, 286.

Kew, mortality from cholera, 193.

Kimberley, 328; proposed sanatorium at, 330; advantages, 331.
Kingston, Mr. Beatty, his pamphlet on combating intemperance, 141.
Klebs, his discovery of the microbe of diphtheria, 184.
Klein, Dr., on diphtheria in cows, 179; in cats, 180.
Koch, Dr., his theory of the bacilli of cholera, 204; on sand-filters, 281.

LAMBETH WATER COMPANY, 194, 277.
Landquart Station, 325.
Latham, Mr. Baldwin, on the supply of water from wells, 299.
Lausen, 282.
Lawrence, Mr., 330.
Lawyers, average duration of life, 69.
Lea river, 193; amount of water supplied from, 277.
Leamington, 345, 347.
Leith Hill, 336.
Leprosy, disinfecting cases of, 244.
Leuk thermal springs, 339.
Lewis, Sir G. C., on the limit of human life, 60.
Lewson, Mrs., 73.
Life assurance companies, records of longevity, 64.
Life, the art of prolonging, 58; duration of, 59, 66; the patriarchs, 62; Greeks and Romans, 63 Middle Ages, 63; assurance companies, 65; three periods of, 75; necessity of occupation, 76.
Linen, use of, 102; its conducting power of heat, 103.
Lister, Sir Joseph, his appeal for funds for the preparation of antitoxin, 163.
Liver, disease of the, 119.
Liverpool, 202.
Llandrindod, 343, 344, 345.
Löffler, his discovery of the microbe of diphtheria, 175, 184.
London, advantages of living in, 11; disadvantages, 12; evidences of "wear and tear," 12; epidemics of diphtheria, 168; number of deaths from, 170; epidemics of cholera, in 1849, 193; in 1854, 194; in 1866, 195; health of, 307.
—— East, Water Company, 277.
—— Water Supply, 272; companies, 277; measures, 283.
Longevity, 58; cases of, 63, 64; conditions favourable to, 66, 74; hereditary, 67; sex, 67; marriage, 68; occupations, 68; moderation in eating and drinking, 70; improbable causes of, 72-74; immoderate use of sugar, 72; means adapted for the attainment, 74; necessity of occupation, 76; exercise of the intellectual faculties, 77; bodily exercise, 79; moderation in food, 83; diet, 84; rules for eating, 85; the use of

alcoholic liquors, 85-87; sleep, 88; warmth, 89; exposure to chills, 89; temperature of the rooms, 90; cleanliness, 90; question of desirability, 92; of total abstinence, 133.

MACKENZIE, DR., 169.

Macnamara, Mr., on the communicability of cholera through drinking water, 197; on badly ventilated rooms, 199; the length of the incubation period, 211.

Macpherson, Dr., his "Bath and Wells of Europe," 316.

Madeira, 333.

Malvern, 345.

Manchester, 291.

Mansfield, Lord, 71.

Margate, 54.

Matjesfontein, 327.

Medical men, average duration of life, 69.

Medical officer of health, 266; duties of, 267.

Mental power, retention of, in old age, 77.

Mental work, result of, 14; various capacities for, 14; monotonous, 16; absence of proper regulations, 17.

Mentone, 333.

Mercury, perchloride of, 257, 260, 263.

Mersey, the, 291.

Metropolis Water Act, 1871, 278, 279.

Micro-organisms of diphtheria, 175; of cholera, 205; the causes of infectious diseases, 234.

Middle Ages, average duration of life in the, 63.

Middlesbrough, 292.

Middlewich, 345.

Milk, a medium of propagating diphtheria, 178, 242.

Mineral waters, 338; thermal, 338; iron, 342; sulphur, 343; salt, 344; alkaline, 345; sulphates of soda and magnesia, 347; carbonates and sulphates of lime and magnesia, 347.

Molesey, 277.

Moritz, St., 343.

Morveau, his work on "The Disinfection of the Air," 243.

Moses, his estimate of the life of man, 62.

Mountain air, effect of, 324; in consumption, 325.

Müller, Dr., 192.

NAIRN, 321.

Nantwich, 345.

Naples, outbreak of diphtheria, 168.

Narcotics, effects of, 30, 88.

National Debt Office, cases of longevity, 64.

Nervous system, effects of alcohol on the, 119.

Neuenahr, 345.

New River Water Company, 277.

Newsholme, Dr., on the rate of mortality from intemperance, 133.

Nice, 322.
North British Life Office, Edinburgh, 65.

OPIUM, effects of, compared with alcohol, 127.
Organisms, minuteness of, 233; cause of infectious diseases, 234; evidence in favour, 235; experiments on anthrax, 236; manner of producing disease, 238; mitigation by cultivation, 239; media for the propagation, 241; existence in water, 301; test by cultivation, 302; removal by filtration, 304.
Over work, diverse opinions on the subject, 13; evidences of, 27.
Oxidation, 291.
Ozone, preparation of, 259.

PACINI, his theory of cholera, 204.
Palmer, William, his refusal of food, 150.
Paris, Children's Hospital, effect of the antitoxin treatment in, 185.
Parkes, Dr., on the exercise of gardening, 82; on rice, 84; on the use of alcohol, 131, 136, 137; on the length of the incubating period in cholera, 211; the influence of oxidation on water, 291; average daily supply, 295; deep wells, 297; the propagation of diseases, 300.
Parliament, the work of members of, 24; disappointing results, 26.
Parr, Thomas, his reputed longevity, 63.
Pasteur, Dr., his researches into organisms, 235, 239.
Paterson, Surgeon-Major General, on the antitoxin treatment, 186.
Patriarchs, longevity of, 62.
Penzance, 321.
Perchloride of mercury, 257, 260, 263.
Permanganate of potassium, 259, 263.
Perspiration, amount of, 106.
Physician, the daily life of a consulting, 22-24.
Plague, the Great, in 1665, lessons from, 3.
Poore, Dr., 107; on animal heat, 102.
Potassium, iodide of, 341; permanganate of, 259, 263.
Priok, 201.
Prisons, insanitary condition of, in 1774, 3.
Prussia, average mortality from diphtheria, 170.
Public Health Act of 1848, 2; amended, 7; of 1875, 267; of 1889, 268.
Püllna, 347.
Pyrmont, 343.

RAIN water, 285.
Ranmore Common, 336.
Ransome, Dr., on the rate of

INDEX.

mortality from intemperance, 133.
Recreation, importance of, 51; forms of, 51.
Redhill, 293.
Rehme, 345.
Rheumatic fever, symptoms of, 222; character of the disease, 224.
Rhodes, Mr. C., his contribution to Kimberley Sanatorium, 330.
Richmond, 328; well, 299.
Riding, advantages of, 43, 81.
River water, quality of, 275, 286.
Rivers Pollution Act, 288, 305, 308.
Riviera, temperature of, 322, 324.
Roberts, Sir W., on the effects of alcohol on digestion, 138, 139.
Romans, duration of life in the time of, 63.
Rooms, disinfection of, 251, 264: *see* Disinfection.
Rothesay, 321.
Roux, M., 184.
Russell, Dr. J. A., on disinfecting woollen articles, 250; washing, 252; carbolic acid, 258.
Rutland, Duchess of, on the best methods of combating intemperance, 141.

SALMON, MR. W., age at his death, 93: *note*.
Salt waters, 344.
Sanitary legislation, 2; progress of, since 1875, 7.
Scarlet fever, symptoms of, 220; infectious character of the disease, 223, 241.
Schwalbach, 343.
Sea air, effects of, 318; bathing, 319; on pulmonary diseases, 321; voyages, 337.
Seaford, 54.
Sewage, methods of dealing with, 288.
Ships, outbreak of cholera on board, 200.
Shoddy, manufacture of, 99-101.
Sicily, outbreak of diphtheria, 168.
Silk, consistence of, 101.
Simon, Sir J., 195.
Sinks, disinfection of, 260.
Slare, Dr., on the use of sugar, 72.
Sleep, quantity of, 40; value, 40, 88; after-dinner, 41; exercise, 43; early rising, 43.
Sleeplessness, symptom of, 29; effects of narcotics on, 30, 88; causes of, 42.
Sloan, Dr., his case of starvation, 155.
Snow, Dr., his theory on the transmission of cholera, 191; on the outbreak in Soho, 197.
Society, its responsibility for the "wear and tear" of life, 37; demands of, 38.
South Downs, 336.
Southwark Water Company, 194, 277.
Spa, 343.
Spaniards, their term for diphtheria, 167.

Spirits, compared with wine, 123; amount of alcohol contained in, 124.
Spirometer, 160.
Splenic fever, 235 : see Anthrax.
Spongy iron, purifying influence of, 265, 282, 305.
Spring water, quality of, 286.
Squire, Dr., on the contagious character of diphtheria, 176.
Starvation, symptoms of, in animals, 146; in human beings, 156.
State, its responsibility for the "wear and tear" of life, 36.
Stockton, 292.
Strathpeffer, 344.
Streatham, 347.
Succi, Signor, his fast, 158; loss of weight, 159; temperature, 160.
Sugar, the use of, conducive to longevity, 72.
Sulphur waters, 343.
Sunbury, 277, 306.
Sydenham, his cases of cholera, 188.

Tanner, Dr., his prolonged fast, 152.
Tannus, 346.
Tea, the use of, 130.
Teddington, 194.
Tees river, 292.
Temperature of the bedroom, 90; of the human body, 95; variations of, 96.
Teplitz thermal springs, 339, 342.
Terebene, 260.

Thames, 193, 194; amount of water supplied from the, 276; alterations, 304; influence of spongy iron, 305.
Thermal waters, 338; baths, 339.
Thermometer, clinical, use of the, 95.
Thoms, Mr., 63; on the records of the life assurance companies, 64; investigations into cases of longevity, 66.
Thorne, Dr., on the transmission of diphtheria through the elementary schools, 177.
Throat, disease of the, 164.
Thymol soap, 264.
Tidy, Dr., on the quality of London water, 284; the result of oxidation, 291.
Tone, want of, 29, 35.
Torquay, 321, 333.
Total abstinence, 133: see Abstinence.
Toulouse, murderer at, his abstention from food, 149.
Tunbridge Wells, 343.
Tynemouth, 320.

United Kingdom Temperance Association, 135.
United States, effect of the antitoxin treatment, 185.

Vaccination, discovery of, 5.
Vals, 346.
Vegetables, increase in the use of, 49.
Ventilation, problem of, 50; of rooms, 253, 261.

INDEX. 363

Ventilators, existence of surface, 172.
Vichy, 345.
Victoria, 328.
Viterbi commits suicide by starvation, 150.

WALES, number of deaths from diphtheria, 170.
Walking, a form of exercise, 81.
Ware, 277.
Water, iced, injurious use of, 49; importance of pure, 212; its use in disinfection, 244; methods of purification, 265; valuable properties, 272; difficulties of supplying, 274; quality of river, 275; amount of consumption, 276; the companies, 277; expenditure, 279; Metropolis Water Act of 1871, 279; reservoirs, 280; filtering beds, 280; duties of the examiner, 282; opinions on the quality, 284; standard of purity, 285; distilled, 285; rain, 285; river or spring, 286; tests, 287; sources of contamination, 288; sewage, 288, 300; floods, 289; purifiying agents, 290; oxidation, 291; exposure to air, 292; two systems of supply, 294; average daily supply, 295; quality of wells, 296; quantity obtainable, 298; propagation of diseases, 299; existence of organisms or germs, 301; test by cultivation, 302; development in filtered or unfiltered, 303; filters, 304; influence of spongy iron, 305; improvement in the quality between 1892 and 1895, 306.
Water Examiner, 280; duties of the, 282.
Waterloo Bridge, 193.
Waterproof clothing, protection of, 108.
Watson, Sir T., 165; on the cause of cholera, 190; the infection of scarlet fever, 241.
"Wear and tear," evidences of, 12; measures against, 36, 40, 50; causes of, 37.
Weber, Dr., on bathing, 319; on the air of the moors, 336.
Wells, quality of the water, 296; supply, 298.
West Middlesex Water Company, 277.
Wight, Isle of, 320.
Wildbad thermal springs, 339, 342.
Wildungen, 348.
Wilks, Dr., on the sedative effects of alcohol, 121, 122; on the beer-drinker, 131; the insurance offices, 134, 135.
Willan, Dr., his case of starvation, 155.
Wind, effect of, 105.
Windows, effect of double, 104.
Wine, moderation in the use of, 49; compared with spirits, 123; amount of alcohol in, 124; influence on digestion, 138.

Wood, Dr., on the increase of insanity, 31.

Wool, an important article of clothing, 98; properties of, 103; power of absorbing water, 106.

Woolwich, the sewers of, 172

YEO, DR. BURNEY, on the temperature of Davos Platz, 326.

Yersin, 184.

ZINC, chloride of, 260, 263.

Zurich, 325.

www.ingramcontent.com/pod-product-compliance
Lightning Source LLC
Chambersburg PA
CBHW020320240426
43673CB00039B/870